"The Matrix is a profoundly useful approach
Simple and direct, it focuses on the most im
through the conceptual clutter—for ACT the...
this way: if you care about ACT, you have to know the Matrix. It's not optional. And
this is the best book yet for learning exactly what it is and how to use it. Highly
recommended."

> —**Steven C. Hayes, PhD**, codeveloper of acceptance and commitment
> therapy (ACT)

"Written in a skillful and highly readable fashion, this volume stands out as a valuable
contribution to ACT practitioners looking for a structured, yet flexible, guide for doing
brief and effective interventions. The authors have succeeded in providing a manual
suitable for private practice, institutional work, and interdisciplinary integration."

> —**Michel. A. Reyes Ortega, PhD**, director of the Contextual Behavioral
> Science and Therapy Institute in Mexico City, Mexico; and clinical
> professor of clinical behavior analysis at the National Institute of
> Psychiatry in Mexico City

"This lively and engaging book provides the most comprehensive, accessible, and practical guide yet to the Matrix model in everyday clinical work. Step by step, the authors
present clear and useful examples of how the Matrix can increase awareness, psychological flexibility, and vitality in adult individuals, couples, and children. *The Essential
Guide to the ACT Matrix* is just that; essential for anyone wishing to understand how to
utilize, and even enjoy, this powerful new clinical tool with their clients."

> —**Christopher McCurry, PhD**, clinical child psychologist in private
> practice, and author of *Parenting Your Anxious Child With Mindfulness
> and Acceptance* and *Working with Parents of Anxious Children*

"This book is the ultimate tool for training psychological flexibility in six basic but
sophisticated steps. Clear guidelines are provided for practicing the ACT Matrix,
present-moment and therapeutic relationship–focused clinical work, getting unstuck,
sharing your own Matrix with clients, and going deeper with each step. Indispensable
for anyone interested in delving more deeply into a functional contextual perspective,
this volume can help clinicians do transformational work with individuals, couples, and
families."

> —**Mavis Tsai, PhD**, cocreator of functional analytic psychotherapy (FAP),
> and research scientist and clinical faculty at the University of Washington

"Tender, yet funny, this book is on the cutting edge of ACT. Offering page after page of practical interventions, newcomers will be presented with a clear frame of reference for doing ACT, and seasoned ACT practitioners will be exposed to fresh material that will excite and invigorate their practice. The six steps presented by the authors are simple, fun, easy to read, and always relevant to working directly with clients. This is my new clinical guide to doing ACT for my students."

—**Timothy Gordon MSW, RSW**, treats attachment and trauma in independent practice in Hamilton, ON, Canada; teaches ACT at McMaster University in the Clinical Behavioural Sciences program; presents workshops around the world; and is renowned for his passion as a presenter, and his experiential approach to training professionals

"For newcomers to ACT or experienced ACT clinicians, this is a much-needed, step-by-step guide to using the Matrix in psychotherapeutic sessions. It places this effective tool right at the heart of the clinical dialogue orienting client's behavioral change. Focused on daily clinical practice, it also illustrates how relational frame theory (RFT), the contextual behavioral approach to understanding human cognition that underlies ACT, can help progressively build better clinical skills and be more helpful to the client. It also extends the application of the Matrix to work with parents and children, couples, and in life coaching. What more could you ask for?"

—**Giovambattista Presti, MD, PhD**, associate professor of psychology, and coordinator of the undergraduate program in psychology at Kore University of Enna in Italy

"Whether you are new to ACT or experienced, you will find real clinical value in this book. As with the Matrix itself, there is nothing extraneous. Everything in it serves the clinician, and by extension the client, in psychotherapy. The writing is engaging and practical. The guidance is clear. The organization of the book is logical. Most compellingly, you will feel immersed in the authors' clinical wisdom and compassion."

—**Gareth Holman, PhD**, coauthor of *Functional Analytic Psychotherapy Made Simple*

The

ESSENTIAL GUIDE

ACT

to the

MATRIX

A Step-by-Step Approach to Using the ACT Matrix Model in Clinical Practice

KEVIN L. POLK, PhD
BENJAMIN SCHOENDORFF, MA, MSc
MARK WEBSTER
FABIAN O. OLAZ, PsyD

CONTEXT PRESS
An Imprint of New Harbinger Publications, Inc.

Publisher's Note

This publication is designed to provide accurate and authoritative information in regard to the subject matter covered. It is sold with the understanding that the publisher is not engaged in rendering psychological, financial, legal, or other professional services. If expert assistance or counseling is needed, the services of a competent professional should be sought.

Distributed in Canada by Raincoast Books

Copyright © 2016 by Kevin L. Polk, Benjamin Schoendorff, Mark Webster, and Fabian O. Olaz
    Context Press
    An imprint of New Harbinger Publications, Inc.
    5674 Shattuck Avenue
    Oakland, CA 94609
    www.newharbinger.com

Cover design by Amy Shoup
Acquired by Tesilya Hanauer
Edited by Jasmine Star
Indexed by James Minkin

Library of Congress Cataloging-in-Publication Data on file

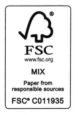
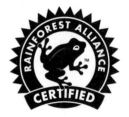

Printed in the United States of America

18   17   16

10   9   8   7   6   5   4   3   2   1   First Printing

"If you want to teach people a new way of thinking, don't bother trying to teach them. Instead, give them a tool, the use of which will lead to new ways of thinking."

—*Buckminster Fuller*

Contents

INTRODUCTION

Training Psychological Flexibility

Acceptance and commitment therapy or training (ACT, pronounced as the word "act") is about doing what works to get where you want to go. It's about choosing your direction and becoming increasingly able to move toward it through your actions, even in the presence of obstacles. Choosing a direction or directions involves identifying who or what is important to you. In ACT, having the ability to choose to do what works in order to move toward who or what is important to you, even in the presence of obstacles, is known as *psychological flexibility*. Over twenty years of international ACT research suggests that psychological flexibility is key to mental health and optimal living. Whereas earlier approaches have focused on how to effectively reduce inner obstacles—unwanted thoughts, feelings, or sensations—ACT seeks to promote valued action even in the face of such obstacles.

In ACT, this is called *valued living*. Valued living is about identifying what's important to us and acting on it, rather than living on autopilot and waiting for obstacles to disappear before doing what's important to us. Valued living means behaving in accordance with our most vital values and goals without allowing our inner experience to function as an obstacle to engaging in actions that can move us toward what really matters. From an ACT perspective, what matters most is not whether we feel good or are able to avoid feeling bad, as pleasant as feeling good may be, and as unpleasant as feeling bad may be. Rather, what matters is having the ability to do things that can effectively move us toward who and what we choose as important to us in life.

In short, the most important things in life generally aren't feeling good or not feeling bad. Though that may at first blush seem strange, consider this easy test. Imagine you could take a pill that would make you feel good and never feel bad again. Would you take it? Most people would. Now imagine this pill had but one little side effect: once you took it, you could never get out of bed or interact with anyone ever again. Would you take it? Surely not. So, if you'd choose not to swallow that pill, it must be because some relationships and things you wish to do are more important to you than feeling good and not feeling bad. ACT is about identifying these valued relationships and endeavors and learning how to effectively move toward them.

How This Book Can Make Training Psychological Flexibility Simpler

This book is a detailed clinical guide to using the ACT matrix, a relatively new way of delivering ACT that aims to simplify the ACT approach and make it more transparent to practitioners and clients alike. In this introduction, we'll present the ACT matrix, including some of its history, and outline a number of key concepts.

Over the past six years, we have worked hard to make ACT, which can at times be complex, both simple and approachable. In this spirit, we've endeavored to keep all discussion of theoretical concepts straightforward enough to be grasped by nonspecialists (though we will, at times, stretch that limit in sections entitled "Going Deeper"). We realize that this means we can't do justice to every subtlety of the model. In a similar vein, although our work is informed by a wealth of clinical and theoretical research into ACT, we'll limit references to a minimum, as this book is first and foremost a guide to matrix-based interventions.

The Matrix

The matrix is a diagram about noticing (see figure 1)—a diagram that can, as it turns out, cue psychological flexibility.

The diagram is composed of two bisecting lines. The vertical line is the experience line. It maps out the difference between the aspects of our experience that come through our five senses—vision, hearing, smell, taste, and touch—and the part of our experience that arises from our mental activity or interoceptive abilities. Here and now, as you read this sentence, see if you can notice the part of your experience that comes through your five senses: the color of the page and the ink, the shapes of the letters, and so on. Then see if you can notice the mental part of your experience: the meaning of the sentence, perhaps some thoughts about where this is leading, and so forth. Now see if you can notice a difference between these two kinds of experience.

The horizontal line is the behavior line. It maps out the difference between actions aimed at moving away from unwanted experience (for example, moving away from fear) and actions aimed at moving toward who or what is important (for example, moving toward a loved one). Take a moment now to recall a time when you did something to move away from fear, and then a time when you did something to move toward a loved one. Can you notice a difference in how it felt to move away and how it felt to move toward?

We believe that, for humans gifted with language, the key to psychological flexibility and valued living is noticing the difference between five-senses and mental experience and noticing the difference between moving toward who or what is important and moving away from unwanted inner experience.

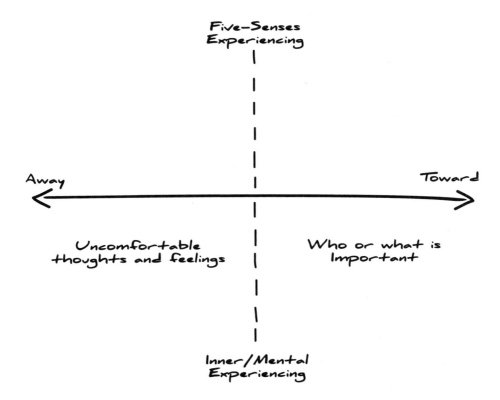

Figure 1.

The matrix invites us to sort our experiences, behavior, and stories into the four quadrants formed by the two bisecting lines. Perhaps you'd like to try it. Draw the two matrix lines on a piece of paper. In the lower right quadrant, write the name of someone important to you. In the lower left quadrant, write one thought, emotion, or memory that can show up and stand in the way of doing something to move toward this important person. In the upper left quadrant, write one thing you can be seen doing when the stuff in the lower left shows up—how you observably either move away from it or act under its control. Finally, in the upper right quadrant, write at least one thing you could be seen doing to move toward this person. Next, step back and notice who chooses that this person is important to you, who can see the stuff that shows up in the lower left quadrant, and who can tell whether what you do is aimed at moving toward this person or away from that stuff at the bottom left. Does what you just mapped out in some way reflect your experience of your relationship with this person?

A Short History of the Matrix

As you can see, the matrix boils down to two lines on a piece of paper. It may seem simple, but it took about seventeen thousand hours between 2004 and the spring of 2009 for Kevin Polk to notice the centrality of noticing those two differences.

During those years, Kevin read broadly on acceptance and commitment therapy, relational frame theory (RFT), and functional contextualism (the philosophy of science upon which RFT and ACT are built), all the while practicing ACT with thousands of clients, mostly in groups. He also spent countless hours discussing ACT, RFT, and functional contextualism with dozens of colleagues—first among them Jerold Hambright and Mark Webster.

Kevin has always had a passion for simplifying complicated topics, and because he enjoys diagramming, through those thousands of hours he was often diagramming ACT processes. Before the introduction of the matrix, ACT had widely been presented through the hexaflex, a hexagon representing six processes central to ACT (Hayes, Strosahl, Bunting, Twohig, & Wilson, 2004). Even though the hexaflex is useful for pointing out processes ACT researchers and clinicians work with, it can feel clinically cumbersome. Kevin, Jerold, and Mark were searching for an alternative diagram, one that they could use when interacting with clients.

In the spring of 2009, Kevin was reading *Derived Relational Responding: Applications for Learners with Autism and Other Developmental Disabilities* (Rehfeldt & Barnes-Holmes, 2009), a book that contains examples of engaging children in sorting tasks to help them acquire verbal abilities, including high-level perspective-taking skills. Think of asking someone to sort a deck of cards according to some criterion, such as color, numbered versus face cards, suit, and so on. Having spent most of his career working with people with trauma memories, Kevin began to think of a trauma memory sorting game. Using index cards, he began playing around with the elements of a trauma memory. First came the sensory experiences that come with the trauma memory, then the way those trauma memories replayed as mental experience. As Kevin stood at a whiteboard and began to draw, two lines showed up: a vertical line with five-senses experience at one end and mental experience at the other, and a horizontal line with attempts to move away from reliving trauma memories at one end and actions to move toward a valued life at the other. Thus the matrix was born.

A trauma memory could now be sorted on the matrix. The first step would be to ask clients to recall the sensory experiences associated with the memory; these are placed at the top of the matrix. The next step would be to ask them to recall some of the uncomfortable inner experiences associated with the trauma memory, like fear; these are placed in the bottom left quadrant. The next step might involve asking clients who or what they might have been moving toward around the time of the trauma; these are placed in the bottom right quadrant. The final step is to ask clients what behaviors they engage in to move away from the fear and other difficult inner experiences; these are placed in the top left quadrant.

Soon Kevin realized that all memories could be sorted this way. Then he realized that all of ACT was about sorting life according to those criteria. Further, sorting experience as "sensory" implies noticing it as different from "inner," and sorting behavior as "toward" implies noticing that it isn't "away." Ultimately, this sorting and noticing of differences puts people in a position to gain perspective on their experience.

Sorting Life Stories

We all have a story to tell—typically a collection of interesting memories. And in the same way that any memory can be sorted into the categories of the matrix, a life story can also be sorted onto the matrix using the four areas created by the two crossed lines. For most members of our highly social species, relationships come first, so we ask "Who is important to you?" before we ask "What is important to you?" We place the answers to those questions in the lower right of the diagram because their importance is in the mind, and people want to move toward them.

A key part of the story is the stuff that can show up inside and get in the way of moving toward who or what is important. Maybe it's the fear that shows up when thinking about asking someone out on a date. These experiences typically go in the lower left quadrant because they are inner experiences that we tend to want to move away from.

Of course, the story also includes behaviors that everyone can see: walking, talking, sitting, and such. These go into the upper two sections of the diagram. First we ask about the behaviors done to move away from unwanted experience, like running away from fear. These are sorted into the upper left quadrant. Finally, we ask about the behaviors that are done, or could be done, to move toward who or what is important. These are sorted into the upper right quadrant.

Sorting on the matrix can help all of us conceptualize our life and notice whether what we do tends to be more in the service of moving toward or moving away. Based on this, we can choose to change or persist in our behavior as needed to move toward what we most care about.

What Is the Matrix Good For?
Absolutely Everything!

You might have recoiled at the boldness of the preceding heading. Yet ACT is a transdiagnostic model based on a radically pragmatic point of view wherein even the use of traditional diagnostic categories is seen through the lens of whether they get us where we want to go. From an ACT perspective, effective treatment doesn't hinge on seeing most mental and behavioral health problems as diseases. It's more useful to determine which processes are most effective in helping people live optimally and which processes keep them stuck, restricting their behavioral options and draining meaning and vitality from their lives. Ultimately, people get stuck when their attempts to move away from unwanted inner experience (like fear) or their behaviors under the control of inner experience (like needing to be right) keep them from doing what's important to them (like building and nurturing relationships, training for and flourishing in an occupation they value, or engaging in vital leisure and self-care activities). Therefore, it is often more useful to look at psychopathology dimensionally—considering the extent to which people get stuck, and in which domains—rather than categorically, with a focus on which precise kinds of inner experience or behavior cause people to get stuck. The matrix can supercharge the transdiagnostic nature of ACT by providing practitioners and clinical and subclinical client populations alike with a common frame of reference: two bisecting lines on a piece of paper.

As for scientific evidence, given that the matrix is a clinician-developed tool, it didn't benefit from much research support early on. This is changing rapidly, and we are aware of a number of research teams worldwide investigating the matrix and using it to good effect. As of this writing, data has been gathered and presented about some of this research (Reyes, 2015; Reyes, Vargas, & Miranda, 2015), and a number of scientific articles are being written up.

ACT's Six Flexibility Processes

Traditionally, ACT has focused on six processes that combine to promote psychological flexibility: cognitive defusion, acceptance, committed action, values, contact with the present moment, and self-as-context.

Cognitive defusion is the ability to distance yourself from your thoughts and feelings so they don't necessarily control your behavior. For example, if like many people you fear public speaking, before giving a presentation you may notice anxiety welling up in your chest and throat, along with thoughts that you can't stand what you feel, you won't be able to speak, and you'd better call in sick. If you take these feelings and thoughts literally—if you fuse with them—they may come to control your behavior, and you might indeed cancel your talk. By gaining a bit of distance and noticing your thoughts as just thoughts and your feelings as just feelings—by defusing from them—you may see that it's possible to give your presentation, even with those thoughts and feelings, which brings us to another ACT process: acceptance.

Acceptance is the ability, once you've gained some distance from your sticky thoughts and feelings, to make space for them and do what is important for you to do, rather than giving up on your goals and engaging in actions aimed at reducing or changing your thoughts and feelings (like calling in sick to move away from the fear and thoughts that you won't be able to speak in public). Acceptance allows you to do what is important to you, leading us to the ACT process known as committed action.

Committed action is simply behavior undertaken to move toward who or what is important to us, even in the presence of obstacles. This brings us to a fourth ACT process: values.

Values are highly individualized. In ACT parlance, "values" refers to how we choose and hold important the people, things, and ways of being that matter to us in life. In our example, values would encompass why it's important to you to make the presentation despite your fear of public speaking.

Contact with the present moment is a process of noticing whatever shows up in the moment—not just thoughts and feelings, but also bodily sensations, what you can perceive with your five senses, and whatever else may show up in the moment. Continuing with the same example, contact with the present moment may help you notice that your thoughts and feelings regarding the presentation sometimes change, as do your related bodily sensations and sensory experience.

Self-as-context, sometimes referred to as the observer self, is the final process. This refers to the ability to step back and take a flexible perspective on what you think, feel, perceive, and do. To wrap up our example, taking a flexible perspective may help you notice all the elements of the other five processes, informing your decision about whether to move toward who or what is important to you in giving the presentation or, as the case may be, to cancel the talk. This ability to take a flexible perspective on your experience and behavior is central to ACT. It also lies at the heart of the matrix.

Traditionally, the six core ACT processes have been presented as a hexagon known as the hexaflex (shown in figure 2). The hexaflex offers a good conceptual description of how ACT works. Of course, there's a big difference between concepts and actions. And when people, clinicians included, are stuck, they rarely need concepts; they need skills. Because the matrix largely bypasses the conceptual step while reaching and activating more basic processes, it can offer a quick and effective way to train ACT skills.

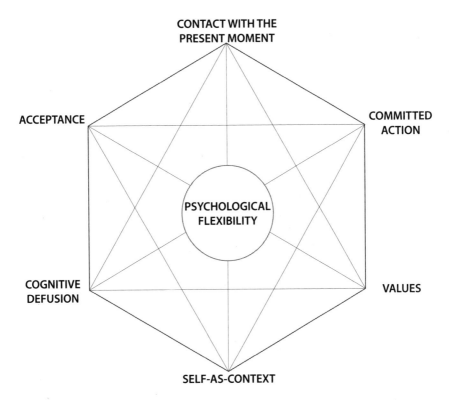

Figure 2.

Appetitive and Aversive

The difference between toward and away moves encompasses a very basic process. In the animal kingdom, behavior serves to move toward things—generally reproductive partners or sources of sustenance, comfort, or fun—or to move away from things: typically threats to physical integrity or survival, such as predators or life-threatening environments. When animal behavior is about moving away from something, it is scientifically termed behavior under *aversive control*, and when it is about moving toward something, it is known as behavior under *appetitive control*. In the absence of threats, behavior is mostly about moving toward. We might even say that living things are essentially about moving toward—toward sources of energy and reproductive partners—and that moving away simply comprises a subset of the behaviors that allow living things to move toward metabolizing energy and reproducing. For this reason, appetitive control is extremely powerful—more powerful than aversive control.

With verbal humans, things quickly get more complicated. Language can make it difficult to sort out what to move away from and what to move toward. In particular, we may find ourselves stuck in trying to move away from unwanted feelings, words, or stories—all part of our inner experience. But because values are so appetitive and unwanted inner experience so aversive, when we find ourselves living a life that largely consists of away moves, wherein the focus is on retreating from unwanted experience, life itself starts to feel constrained and stuck and can even become aversive. This can lead to efforts to check out of life or, at the extreme, to end it altogether.

Thankfully, moving toward values is so appetitive that when we find our way to a life largely about those people and things that are important, it brings a sense of freedom and vitality. In ACT terms, psychological flexibility can be thought of as bringing our behavior and our lives under the appetitive control of who and what matter most to us. In this light, the matrix can serve as a road map to a life lived under the appetitive control of your own values.

Language

As you read these words, you are using an amazing ability: language. Language is a wonderful tool for conveying information from one person to another and can be useful in countless ways. Language can also be a problem. Take the thought *I can't do that*. You've probably had it show up at times when you actually could do something, but the thought that you couldn't stopped you. That's just one of the problems with language. Another is fear. Of course, fear isn't language; it's a feeling that shows up in the presence of danger, perhaps a lion, tiger, or bear. However, thanks to language and the ability it gives us to link our inner experience with mental images, we can experience a similar level of fear at an imagined situation, like simply thinking of asking someone out on a date. Language lets us go into the future and imagine the other person saying no, leading to a present fear of rejection. If the fear based on this imagined scenario is strong enough, we might restrict our behavior and not ask the person out.

Countless little scenarios can play out in the mind and restrict a person's behaviors. And there might be just as many scenarios that can open that same person up. ACT takes a close look at how language and "thinking" (the act of producing strings of words) function in our lives. Our words are always taking us somewhere. When we notice this process, we're in a better position to determine whether our language is getting us where we want to go or whether we're struggling with the unwanted aspects of it.

A Bit About Relational Frame Theory

Saying that the human capacity to produce words can either restrict or open behavior calls for a theory of how that happens—hopefully one that's useful for helping people open up and adopt more varied behaviors. The theory also needs to show how the products of language get people stuck. ACT scientists have developed just such a theory: relational frame theory (RFT). We aren't going to try to explain RFT in this book; we'll just take a quick look at RFT and point out some of the RFT underpinnings in how we use the matrix, as well as try to speak in ways that are consistent with the theory, to the best of our ability and to the extent that doing so may be useful to you in your work and interventions. For a further treatment of the links between the matrix and RFT, please refer to "Under the Hood: Basic Processes Underlying the Matrix" (Schoendorff, Webster, & Polk, 2014), and for a highly readable introduction to RFT, refer to *Learning RFT* (Törneke, 2010).

A fair amount of RFT is about how sensory experience is transformed into words. Take the word "lemon," for example. As you experienced lemons in early life, you added the frames "yellow," "sour," "juicy," and so forth to the sound "lemon" until finally, as you said the word "lemon," those frames showed up in your experience. In a way, you became a bit fused (restricted) in your experiencing of lemons, but that works because it's handy to know your experience of lemons. However, this can be taken too far. Let's say that once you became ill after eating a lemon, so now you frame "illness" with "lemon." Then, in the future when you see a recipe that needs a bit of lemon, you might say, "Never! I *hate* lemons. I will never use lemons." You can see how your future behavior (using lemon in a recipe) might be limited by your previous framing of the word "lemon" with illness.

Words are usually used within sentences, and those sentences often come together to form stories. In this way, certain words can become a part of a story that keeps people stuck—for example, "I don't use lemons because they made me sick in the past." If you stick with that story, you'll narrow your culinary choices.

Let's take this a little further. Say you hear that Judy likes lemons. The "Judy" frame becomes part of your lemon story. And say Judy once lied to you. Now the frame "lied" is also part of your lemon story. This may lead you to something you never thought before: *People who like lemons are not to be trusted.* As a result, you might become uncomfortable around people who like lemons, and that might limit your behavior around them.

Forming these kinds of connections is known as *derived relational responding*. It is *derived* because its functions and consequences are not contained in five-senses experience. It is *relational* because the derivation is a result of relating, or framing, one set of words or inner experiences with another set of words or inner experiences. And it is *responding* because it leads to a response: a toward or an away behavior resulting from this framing.

We all engage in derived relational responding, all the time. We humans tend to be fearful and cautious, so it's easy for us to take something neutral, like plain old lemons, associate it with something unpleasant, like illness, and then add a frame of distrust related to Judy's lying. And voilà! Distrust is caught up with our hate of lemons.

Of course, some behavioral limitations, such as what not to do at a formal dinner, come in handy. Others, like our lemon story, are wacky and limiting but not particularly problematic. Then there are those that can become problematic. We may stop going to certain places because of a story that says it's dangerous when it isn't dangerous at all. We may not apply for a job because of a story that says we're going to be rejected anyway. The human mind has a seemingly infinite ability to take uncomfortable stuff like fear and add it to stories that then restrict what we do. And because the mind is infinitely better at adding than subtracting, it's all too easy to get caught in a cycle of heaping more "stuck" framing onto stories. In the next paragraph, we'll unpack how this might work.

Relational frame theory describes how the mind is, at root, additive. Our higher or verbal cognitive functions are dominated by a process through which we can put a number of mental experiences in relation with one another, the coherence of which relations we can then track out in the world of five-senses experience. This allows us to assess if things are heavier or lighter, bigger or smaller, scarier or less scary, and so on, and then behave accordingly. In this process, subtracting mental experiences is extremely difficult. See for yourself: For the next thirty seconds, try not to think of a purple unicorn…

Once you experience this thought and as you seek to push it away, it tends to persist. It's much easier to think of additional things than to not think of something. You can check that out now by trying to add other things to your thoughts of the purple unicorn.

When we orient our behavior not just in relation to our five-senses experience but also more broadly, such as in relation to who or what is important to us, the process of framing can either get us stuck or help us get unstuck and flexibly move toward who or what is important. The way we frame the situations we experience—through comparing, assessing, judging, explaining, and reasoning—can either increase or decrease flexibility, and multiply or decrease our options and choices.

For clinicians, using relational frame theory involves noticing whether what we do and say, and what clients do and say, adds framing that promotes or inhibits flexibility in a given situation. When we attend to this, the end result will be more workable actions from clients—actions that help them move in valued directions.

Getting Unstuck

Distilling the preceding sections, a key aim of ACT is adding flexible framing to stuck stories. If the mind were mechanical, we could simply remove stuck frames in order to restore flexibility—for example, removing the pesky "lie" framing from the lemon story. If you've tried this, you may have noticed that it doesn't work very well. The more likely result is adding yet another frame, "trying to remove lying from lemons," to lemons. This is what happens when we try not to think of something; we just think about it all the more. So in ACT, we focus on adding more flexible framing instead—in other words, adding framing that can expand behaviors rather than restrict them.

The good news is, teaching people more flexible framing is both easy and fun. Just start sorting stuck stories, or parts of stories, into the matrix, then step back and look at the story to add the "big picture" frame. There are many, many more ways to promote more flexible framing around stories, but the basic act of sorting the elements of a story into the quadrants of the matrix allows framing from a distance, which readily reveals that, in every situation, there are more potential responses than we can initially notice. That kind of distancing framing is also known as perspective or deictic framing, and it is at the heart of the matrix's effectiveness. It allows us to choose how to respond or behave, bringing us to another very important part of the matrix: noticing workability.

Noticing Workability

As noted earlier, ACT is built on the functional contextual point of view, which is possibly better understood as the workability point of view. *Workability* simply means noticing whether behaviors work to move us in a chosen direction. In ACT, these directions are called values. A central question when using the matrix is "Who or what is important to you?" If we know who or what is important to us, we can notice whether our behaviors work to move us toward the life we'd like to be leading. In terms of the matrix, we notice this primarily through our five-senses experience. Did our behavior make the difference we sought to make? We also notice it through our inner experience. Did it work to give us a sense that we behaved like the person we want to be, in line with who or what is important to us?

You might have noticed that we used the word "notice" in regard to workability. We purposely didn't refer to analyzing whether behaviors are working. What's the difference? Analyzing uses verbal reasoning to determine workability. But it's words that get people stuck in the first place. So although verbal reasoning might work for determining workability, biases can enter into such an analysis.

When we say "noticing," we refer to the type of noticing you do when riding a bicycle. While balancing, you aren't doing a verbal analysis of balancing. That's much too slow to be useful as you adjust your behaviors to maintain balance. Noticing whether behaviors work to move us toward our values is much the same. Obviously, some of the biases inherent in language are still present, influencing whether a given behavior feels like more of a toward move than an away move. But by merely noticing rather than judging and evaluating, we get closer to letting go of words and allowing experience to be our guide.

Letting go of words and instead relying on our experience is central to getting unstuck, but this is a tricky game that never stops. We are surrounded by words. Almost every waking moment, words are in our midst and in our minds. Even in sleep, our dreams deliver words, along with images. This verbal soup that we swim in is all too easy to get caught up in, landing us back in verbal analysis. You might wonder, *Am I on the right path? Am I saying the right things? Am I doing the right things?* These and a thousand other questions come to mind, demanding an answer, as if we had foreknowledge of exactly what does and doesn't work.

Obviously, verbal learning can provide some helpful guidelines for how to behave: to get out of bed in the morning and start putting one foot in front of the other to get the day rolling; to engage in work or other activities that offer opportunities for identifying workable behaviors. But how to optimally fine-tune our behavior isn't something we can absolutely know in advance. Therefore, it's better to be in the moment and notice what works and what doesn't. Be forewarned: The verbal mind wants nothing to do with such experiencing. It wants absolutes, and under its influence, letting go can seem impossible. However, it's really no more difficult than letting go of a rope in a gentle game of tug-of-war in which neither party is pulling that hard. Letting go simply means regaining balance after a moment. Of course, letting go of a rope is a physical thing, whereas letting go of words is an inner experience. And with that, we enter the tradition of thousands of years of meditation and mindfulness practice.

Mindfulness Without "Mindfulness"

The creators of ACT didn't invent something new when they started working with the notion that words can be a problem. Buddhists arrived at the same conclusion over two thousand years ago. Essentially all meditation and mindfulness traditions have in some way or another embraced the practice of letting go of words or the results of words. For example, while sitting and being mindful, you might notice the words "I'm not very good at being mindful" showing up. If you buy those words or get hooked by them, a battle to get better at mindfulness will probably ensue—which wouldn't result in better mindfulness. So mindfulness traditions provide suggestions along the lines of "Notice the words go floating by." That "floating by" quality speaks to letting go of the effects of words.

Unfortunately, although mindfulness practice may be beneficial for most people, only a small fraction of the human population engages in it. The rest of humanity is caught up with words, buying into words, fighting with words, and so on. ACT has emphasized mindfulness practices in the hopes that people would take them up. Then, by combining mindfulness with defusion and acceptance techniques, they could get out of their minds and into their lives—to paraphrase the title of a popular ACT book (Hayes, 2005). As you might imagine, even with the prompting of therapists, teachers, and others offering ACT, most clients never manage to turn mindfulness into an ongoing practice, and those who don't are left out of the game a bit.

Developing the matrix approach was, in large part, a by-product of our efforts to find a way to help people who don't or won't engage in mindfulness practice get into a mindful space. Many ACT practitioners were already using the word "notice" as a way of prompting mindfulness without explicitly invoking formal mindfulness practice. The matrix diagram took this to a new level because it's visual as well as verbal. Throughout this book, we refer to showing clients the matrix and pointing to it, along with using words to describe the processes involved. The words invite people to notice common experiences that tend to be easy to notice. They are the fingers pointing at the moon of experiencing. Sensory and mental experiencing are readily available, as are the experiences of how it feels to move toward and how it feels to move away. Answering many matrix-related questions is also easy, including where to sort verbal material into the matrix. It's all fairly easy, and it's all mindful at the same time—and mindfulness need never be mentioned.

A Stance That Says, "Yes, And..."

Developing and training psychological flexibility isn't about fighting against anything, least of all against the mistakes that inevitably come with learning. It's about working and moving toward who or what is important. If you learn only one thing from this book, we hope that it will be to take an open stance toward everything that shows up. Human minds are highly trained in noticing what's wrong and commanding us to move away from mistakes and wrongness. They tend to shout, *No! Don't think, feel, or do this or that.* A cornerstone of ACT is that this tendency of the mind plays a large role in getting us stuck and can cause even the best therapeutic approaches to grind to a halt if the client, therapist, or both remain mired in this unwinnable struggle.

This book proposes a stance that welcomes everything that shows up—thoughts, emotions, memories, behavior—with a gentle "Yes, and..." The "Yes" validates whatever shows up, and then the "and..." gently reorients attention toward whatever else may be present, possible, or hoped for. Helping clients develop psychological flexibility thus begins with your stance as a therapist and ends when they can adopt this stance and adapt it to their circumstances in the service of moving toward the life they want.

About This Book

Throughout this book we'll show you various ways you can use the matrix to help your clients and yourself get unstuck and moving toward valued living. This book is an intervention manual. It presents a step-by-step approach to delivering ACT that has been adapted and implemented across varied populations and contexts. Although the matrix evolved to treat clinical populations in groups, it quickly adapted to individual treatment. Then it started mutating and spreading to broader populations and contexts: couples, families, schools, organizations, and communities (Polk & Schoendorff, 2014). In this book, you'll learn to use ACT with the matrix in ways that you can easily adapt to your own practice and the populations you serve. You need not be a clinician to profit from this book; it can also enhance any coaching practice or workplace intervention.

Part 1 of the book details six basic steps for working with the matrix. Each step can generally be covered in one session, and we often do so. However, the process set forth in part 1 is an approach that can be used flexibly, in keeping with the very flexibility it encourages. In part 2 of the book, we turn to how to use the matrix to work on relationships and in the social realm: in the context of the therapeutic relationship; with couples, families, and children; and in coaching. (For guidance on using the matrix for team building and with work groups, see Seys, 2014, and Polk, 2014, respectively.) Part 2 also takes a brief look at integrating the matrix with approaches other than ACT.

To get the most out of this book, initially try to practice the steps as closely to the way we present them as you can. At the end of each of the chapters in part 1, presenting the six basic steps, you'll find a practice checklist. Use it. The steps have been honed by our clinical and training experience. The more closely you practice them as they are outlined, the more likely you are to experience—and let your clients experience—their power. You'll then be in a better position to adapt the approach to your own practice and style.

The reason why we're outlining the importance of using the exercises as we present them has to do with the power of language. We've fine-tuned these exercises to increase the probability that they will quickly engender greater psychological flexibility in your clients—and you. If you start adding lots of other language around them, you may inadvertently add frames that diminish their power.

For each step in part 1 of the book, we include recommended home practices for clients. We encourage you to do all of these practices yourself, engaging with the material just as your clients will. We are, after all, swimming in the same soup. Doing these practices for yourself will enhance your ability to understand clients' experiences with the matrix, both in and out of session. It will also make you a better and more credible instructor. After all, would you choose a surfing instructor who isn't a surfer?

By the way, the checklists for the steps in part 1 of the book, as well as various worksheets we offer, are available for download at http://www.newharbinger.com/33605 (see the back of the book for instructions on how to access them). Feel free to print these materials and use them in your private practice.

A Book About Practicing Basic Moves

By practicing some basic moves, which we present in the six steps of part 1, you'll acquire key skills and develop competencies that will serve you in your professional practice and personal life. These skills will grow as you practice the basic steps, and you'll soon notice increased flexibility in your clinical practice. Once again, this is analogous to developing the skill of balancing as you learn to ride a bicycle. Once you've mastered balancing, the skill of leaning into turns soon shows up, as does the skill of looking at the point you want ride toward.

As you start working with the matrix, you may need or wish to spend more time on some of the basic steps. Don't worry if you initially find yourself devoting a couple of sessions to the material covered in a single chapter. That's perfectly natural and reflects a flexible response to your own learning curve. In addition, some clients may require more deliberate, repeated practice, especially for the basic verbal aikido moves of step 4 or the perspective-taking interview in step 6.

As with learning to ride a bike, working with the matrix looks (and is) simple, yet it isn't easy. So begin by following the steps in order. Also note that it takes a fair amount of practice to become a flexible matrix practitioner. That practice involves deliberate repetition of the steps until you notice that you can use them flexibly in most situations. Then, once you master the skills, you might notice that you begin to improvise in order to ride exactly how you want to and where you want to go.

A Book About Learning in the Present Moment

Learning is a present-moment process. ACT and the matrix are about learning what works to promote valued living. To that end, this book is about training behaviors in the present moment—behaviors that can be taken out on the road to increase valued living for your clients and for yourself.

You've already done a lot of learning in your life. Recall when you were learning to drive a car. Now recall going around your first curve after going full speed on a straight stretch. That was probably challenging. You might have braked too much and braked too little—all in the same curve. Your passengers probably had a rough ride. However, after just a few more curves you were braking appropriately. You learned quickly because you were getting instant feedback from the car. Had you been steering an ocean liner, it would have taken much, much longer, because the feedback from turning an ocean liner might take minutes to show up. You need instant feedback to learn quickly, and that's what we are getting at with the matrix.

Working with the matrix will help your clients be in contact with the broader aspect of the situations they find themselves in and provide them (and you) with almost instant feedback about the usefulness, or workability, of their behaviors in terms of promoting valued living. Said another way, your clients will learn both toward and away moves that work because the matrix will help them stay connected to the present moment. Just like the instant feedback that occurs when learning to brake around a curve, the matrix opens up almost instant feedback about what is and isn't working to promote valued living. It takes a little practice, but the learning comes quickly.

A Book About Practicing a Practice

Functional contextualism, upon which ACT is based, is a pragmatic point of view. With ACT, we are searching for useful ways to help people learn what works to increase valued living in diverse situations and life circumstances. With workability, we aren't focusing on right and wrong; we are simply and pragmatically looking for behaviors that enhance valued living. Functional contextualism is nonjudgmental. Behaviors simply have purposes and work, to a greater or lesser extent, to facilitate valued living. The judgmental terms "good" and "bad" are seldom used within the functional contextual point of view. Functional contextualism holds all categorizations lightly, because the more we try to fit something into a category and keep it there, the more inflexibility shows up. Since all matrix work is targeted at increasing psychological flexibility, a rigid attachment to categories rarely works.

Books are relatively poor tools for learning, especially when it comes to learning a practice. A bike riding manual will only go partway toward helping you actually ride a bike. Learning a new behavior involves practicing the new behavior over and over again, noticing mistakes and possible improvements, practicing again while incorporating these improvements, and then noticing new mistakes and potential improvements. There is something circular to optimal learning, and the linear form of a book doesn't do it justice. In this book, we have sometimes deliberately risked appearing repetitive. The aim is not to bore you, but to gently and continuously reorient you to the practice as you learn its basic steps.

In the end, practicing the six basic steps of matrix work is the most useful thing you can do. Just as with practicing driving, playing the guitar, or playing tennis, magic happens when you practice the basics. For now, let's turn our attention to chapter 1 and the first basic step in working with the matrix.

PART 1

The Six Basic Steps

The first part of this book outlines six steps for increasing psychological flexibility. As mentioned in the introduction, each step can generally be covered in one session. However, as you become more proficient in training your clients in the skills outlined in these chapters, you'll probably notice that you can combine them in a flexible way to suit the needs and pace of each client and to resonate with your own personal style.

In each of these chapters, we'll first describe how to conduct that step in session. Then we'll set forth the home practice you can invite clients to engage in to reinforce in-session learning. Of course, human nature being as it is, therapy doesn't always proceed neatly, so each chapter in part 1 includes a section on potential traps to watch out for and how to flexibly sidestep them. Toward the end of each chapter in part 1, you'll find answers to some frequently asked questions about the material in that chapter. Each chapter concludes with a section entitled "Going Deeper," in which we discuss some of the underlying processes and strategies that lie at the heart of matrix work without necessarily being part of what we tell clients. Although you can probably use the matrix perfectly competently without reading these parts, you may be interested in understanding some of the foundations of the work. Finally, at the end of each chapter you'll find a checklist to guide you in applying that step as you begin this work. In time, the sequence will become second nature, and you'll also begin to fine-tune your approach to reflect your therapeutic style and to address the needs of individual clients.

CHAPTER 1

Step 1: Setting Up the Point of View

The first step in using the matrix is setting up the psychological flexibility point of view as the context in which the work—whether therapy or training—will take place, which also serves to prime people to start using this point of view in their lives. All matrix work is aimed at getting people to notice the matrix outside of session. After all, life happens outside of therapy, and this is where people will ultimately experience the full effectiveness of the matrix point of view.

In this chapter we outline a way to present the matrix and establish the psychological flexibility point of view, generally in a single session. This is just one of many potential ways to present it. We suggest that you practice the approach outlined here a few times to give yourself a chance to experience the various aspects of establishing this point of view.

Making Matrix Work Safe and Fail-Safe

Before we describe this first step, we'll introduce a few principles of matrix conversation skills that we've found central to this work.

When working with the matrix, your first task is to create a safe and interesting environment in which people can learn to interact differently with their experiences and behaviors. The primary stance involves never making people feel that they're failing at the skills you're inviting them to practice. Of course, different people will respond differently to what you present to them and show varying degrees of skill. Mistakes will be made, both by you and by your clients, and mistakes are actually a valuable part of learning. So the key is to create an environment in which it's safe to make mistakes and in which they're seen as a normal part of learning. We believe that people's behavior in a given context is a function of their learning history and abilities. In this sense, behavior is never wrong; indeed, from a functional contextual point of view it is only workable or not—including the behavior of pointing out mistakes. Most likely, a behavior is present because it proved useful in some way in the past. So instead of necessarily trying to point out mistakes, we've found it most workable not to struggle with clients—notably every time we notice struggling with a client.

Behavior takes place in context, and in its context it is always right in the sense that it is a function of that context. In the matrix, context comprises what people contact through five-senses experience and through inner experience and includes the whole of their learning history. Therefore, behavior can only change when something changes in one or more of these aspects of the context.

The inner context is largely experienced in the form of stories, which can both drive and obscure behavior. When these stories are inflexible, behavior can become unworkable, and it can also be more difficult to bring into view its broader consequences on one's life. The matrix helps people sort their experience and stories in such a way that stories, behavior, and consequences become more apparent and come into sharper focus, allowing people to identify whether their behavior is workable. The psychological flexibility point of view is about perspective-taking skills, and the matrix is an avenue for developing them.

One of the main skills in matrix work is what we call "yessing." Yessing is a word we've coined to denote the practice of never contradicting clients and instead beginning responses with the words "Yes, and…" As you'll see, what usually comes next are words that aim to point to some aspect of clients' experience, bringing their experience into perspective and, often, inviting them to notice a difference.

Whenever we work with the matrix, we make sure clients never fail, whether at sorting with the matrix, at home practice, or at noticing their experience. When we keep the context safe in this way, clients readily turn toward engaging in matrix work.

Working with the matrix can be likened to practicing a verbal form of aikido—a Japanese martial art also known as "the way of love." The principles of aikido involve aligning with another person's energy and redirecting it instead of blocking it. Aikido practice emphasizes being present in the moment, taking whatever is offered by an opponent or partner, and avoiding struggle. Practicing verbal aikido through the matrix involves taking clients' words and directing them into the matrix, thereby inviting them to sort their stories and behavior. As with aikido, proficiency in verbal aikido requires repeated and deliberate practice. We will provide many opportunities for such practice in this book and invite you to practice these client exercises for yourself. Another important aspect of aikido is that it is based on a principle of equality, with practitioners at all levels practicing together. The ACT approach mirrors this, being grounded in a sense of radical equality. In ACT, we are all in the same boat, practitioners and clients alike. (Chapter 4 presents yessing and verbal aikido in greater depth.)

Asking Clients What Brings Them to You

From the get-go, you can set up therapy as a context of choice. This helps create a safe space for clients. Offering choices is a reliable antecedent to behavior, and choices are largely appetitive for most people.

The first choice you can offer clients is about how to structure the first session. Offer to spend a bit of time on what brings them to therapy, then ask whether you can present a point of view that people have found useful for helping them do what's important even in the presence of obstacles. Finally, offer to make time for questions and comments before inviting clients to choose whether they want to engage in this work with you. Then, before you move on, ask if they'd like to structure their time in this way or in some other way.

One you get permission, you can move to asking what brings your client to therapy, which you might phrase as follows.

Therapist: Tell me what brings you here. As you do, can I interrupt to ask questions? I'll only ask questions that will help me get how it feels for you to experience what brings you here. Once I have a sense that I get it—in broad outline, of course, not in every detail—I'll reflect it back to you. Then one of three things can happen. You may say, "Yes, that's pretty much it." Or you may say, "That's pretty much it, but there are a couple more things." Or you may say that I didn't get it at all, in which case I hope you'll give me a second chance. Then, once you feel that I get it, I'll show you a point of view we could work with. Are you okay with that?

In the conversation that ensues, ask about the impacts of what clients are experiencing. How does it affect their relationships, work or studies, leisure activities, and self-care? Be sure you take the time to do that, since not taking the time to connect with and validate their experience often causes people to get stuck and become unreceptive to attempts to help. Once clients recognize your reflection of their experience and sense that you get where they're at, they'll feel validated and heard. They'll also be more open to looking at whatever you want to show them. This sets the stage for presenting the psychological flexibility point of view.

Introducing the Matrix

The matrix is, at root, a way to present and work within a functional contextual point of view, which we'll refer to variously as the point of view, the psychological flexibility point of view, or the matrix. The terminology matters less than making sure we operate from this perspective.

We've found that there's no need to begin by talking about what the point of view is. Rather, we socialize clients into it by helping them take a first peek through the matrix. So ask clients if they'll let you show them a point of view. If they say yes, you can then proceed along the following lines.

Therapist: This is just a point of view. I don't claim that it's the only possible point of view, the best point of view, or even an accurate representation of reality. It's simply a point of view that people have found makes it easier to choose to do what's important, even in the presence of obstacles. When we look through this point of view at an animal, say a rabbit, at any given time we can see it either moving toward things that can be perceived with the five senses, such as carrots or other rabbits, or moving away from things that can be perceived with the five senses, such as barking dogs. Sometimes we can even see rabbits moving toward carrots while moving away from barking dogs.

As you say these words, draw a horizontal line on a piece of paper, put arrowheads at each end, and write the word "toward" to the right and the word "away" to the left. (You can also use a whiteboard for this, but if you do, you'll want to document the final, filled-in matrix, perhaps photographing it with your phone and with the client's.)

Then begin to address how this dynamic applies to humans, saying something along the following lines.

Therapist: We humans are similar to rabbits in that we can also be seen to move toward or away from things that can be perceived with our five senses, such as carrots and dogs. But I don't imagine you came here because you're all about carrots or because of a paralyzing fear of barking dogs. That's where the stuff below the horizontal line comes in. We humans can also be seen moving toward people and things that are important to us and that can't always be perceived with our five senses. And we can also be seen moving away from things that can't be perceived with our five senses, like fear or difficult thoughts or memories. So now let's see if we can take a first look at this point of view from your own perspective.

At this point, draw a vertical dotted line bisecting the horizontal line. With practice, you may start to leave a space in the middle of both lines.

Next, begin to guide your client's first exploration of the matrix with five key questions:

Who and what are important to you?

What shows up and gets in the way of moving toward who or what is important?

Who stands at the center of the point of view?

What are some of the things you do to move away from unwanted inner stuff?

What do you do or could you do to move toward who or what is important?

Who and What Are Important?

Begin by asking, "Who is important to you?" Then ask, "What is important to you?" You can also write "Who and what are important?" in the lower right quadrant of the matrix if you like. It's important to first focus on who is important, because nearly everyone will name someone, and you want clients to succeed. Common answers include spouse, children, coworkers, and friends. Next, ask what life domains and other things are important to clients. Common answers include work, learning, health, personal growth, being in nature, and having fun. As clients answer, write or have them write their responses in the lower right quadrant. In many cases, both questions—who and what—will elicit responses that reflect clients' values. And in fact, we do sometimes ask "Who and what is important to you?" This phrasing works fine when speaking with clients, and we encourage you to use it if you wish. In this book, we'll stick with "who or what is important" for grammatical reasons, even though it doesn't quite capture our intent.

While we're on language, we'd like to share that although we use the word "values" in some descriptive parts of this book, we rarely if ever use it with clients, as we've found that the word can at times be sticky and send clients into their head. We've found that referring to who or what is important when we want to point to values is often a more effective way to help clients contact their values. This may be due to the fact that the word "important" is more general and less conceptual than the word "values." In fact, with clients, we rarely use other conceptual terms from the traditional ACT vocabulary, such as defusion, acceptance, commitment, compassion, and mindfulness. This is because we like to stick as close to clients' language as possible and also because, in our experience, people who are stuck rarely need concepts explained to them—they need training in the skills that will get them unstuck.

To ensure clients don't fail, and to keep this first peek through the matrix appetitive, pay attention to their pace. As long as they name one important person, they can start looking through this point of view. So if they seem stumped after naming just one or two people or things, you can say, "Good sample! We're not trying to be complete here; we're just taking a first look through this point of view. As we come back to it later, you may notice other people or things that are important to you." This initial foray into the matrix is more about getting clients to successfully look through the point of view than it is about what they see as they first peek through it.

What Shows Up and Gets in the Way?

At this point, ask clients whether they notice that they always—every second of every minute of every day—do things to move toward who or what is important to them. When in all probability they answer no, you can express relief that you aren't alone and then say something like "If we don't always do the actions that would move us toward who or what is important, it must be because there are obstacles, right?" Then describe how, from this point of view, there can be two kinds of obstacles. One is outside obstacles, such as physical distance, which can prevent us from spending more time with loved ones who live far away. Acknowledge that outside obstacles are important and mention that you'll look at them later. Then turn to inner obstacles: thoughts, emotions, bodily sensations, memories, and other internal experiences that can show up and get in the way of doing what would move us toward who or what is important. You could use fear as an example, or perhaps guilt, which can stand in the way of calling loved ones who live far away.

Then ask, "What shows up and gets in the way of moving toward who or what is important to you?" You can also write this in the lower left quadrant, if you like, streamlining to just "What shows up and gets in the way?" Typical responses include anger, sadness, depression, and anxiety. Other responses include thoughts, such as "I can't do this" or "I'm not good enough." We like to put thoughts in quotation marks to denote them as thoughts. Again, record clients' responses on the matrix, placing them in the lower left quadrant. Keep the conversation light and flowing. It's not about being all-encompassing at this point. When the pace slows, say something like "That's a pretty good sample for a first look. We don't have to be comprehensive. We'll have plenty of time to look at this in more detail later."

Who Is at the Center of the Point of View?

At this point, turn to clients and, pointing in turn to each of the lower quadrants, ask, "Who can choose and notice who or what is important to you, and who can notice the inner stuff that shows up and gets in the way?" It might take some gentle coaching, but most clients will readily answer "me." Then draw a circle at the intersection of the two lines and say something like "Yes. Only you can choose and notice who or what is important to you and notice what can show up and get in the way. So I'll write 'Me noticing' at the center of the point of view and circle it, because you're at the center of the point of view, and in our work together, we'll be sure to keep you there." (This step is depicted in figure 3.)

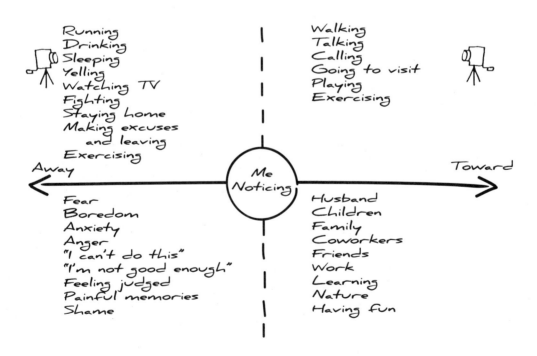

Figure 3.

What Do You Do to Move Away from Unwanted Inner Stuff?

Before moving on, let clients know that you're moving to the upper part of the matrix. In the lower part you were talking about stuff no one else can see, like thinking and feeling. Say that the upper part is about what everyone can see us do.

Ask, "What can you typically be seen doing to move away from, or under the control of, that unwanted stuff that shows up inside of you?" If you like, write that question in the upper left quadrant, streamlining it to just "What can you be seen doing to move away?" You could give an example, like "To move away from fear, some people might hide." Typical responses include running, drinking, avoiding, sleeping, yelling, and fighting. As you or your clients record these responses on the matrix, leave about an inch of free space to the left of the vertical line. You'll need it for step 2 (see chapter 2).

We draw a little camera at the far end of the upper left quadrant to orient clients toward behavior that can be seen, because people may initially find it difficult to describe observable behavior. Stories often show up and get in the way. These stories seldom focus on behavior; more commonly, they involve explanations or conceptual names for behavior. For example, people may say "avoiding" or name some psychological concept, such as self-sabotaging, rather than saying "staying home" or "making excuses and leaving." Use gentle prompting when this happens, asking, "And what do you usually do when you're avoiding? What can you be seen doing when you avoid?" If clients still can't name observable behavior, just write down what they said and move on. Remember, it's more about sorting than about sorting right.

What Can You Do to Move Toward Who or What Is Important?

Finally, ask, "And what can you be seen doing—or what could you be seen doing—to move toward who or what is important to you?" If you like, write a streamlined version of this question in the upper right quadrant. Typical responses include walking, talking, calling, visiting, and playing. As you or your clients write these down, leave about half an inch of free space to the right of the vertical line. Again, you'll need that space in step 2.

It isn't uncommon for the same behavior to show up on both sides: for example, sleeping or exercising. If this happens or you feel that this may be the case, you could say, "So you've noticed doing this (*pointing to the behavior*) as an away (*or toward*) move. And you've also noticed doing it as a toward (*or away*) move." Or, alternatively, "Have you ever noticed doing it as a toward (*or away*) move?" Then ask, "When you do this, who can tell whether you're doing it as an away or a toward move?" Clients seldom require much coaching to notice that they are best placed to notice that. You can then conclude by saying, "You truly stand at the center of this point of view, because only you can choose and notice who or what is important to you, what inner stuff can show up and get in the way, and whether what you do is a toward move or an away move."

Agreeing on Flexible Therapeutic Objectives

Now that clients have taken their first peek through the matrix, you can say something like "That's the point of view." If you wish, you can say the matrix is also called the psychological flexibility point of view. Then, before moving on, say something along the following lines.

Therapist: I only need to ask you two more questions to wrap up this initial exploration and see if you'd be willing for us to work from this point of view. Imagine that you could choose between two possible lives: life number one, here on the left (*pointing to the left side of the matrix*), in which what you do is mostly, though not exclusively, about moving away from this kind of stuff (*pointing to the bottom left*); and life number two, here on the right (*pointing to the right side of the matrix*), in which what you do is mostly, though not exclusively, about moving toward who or what is important to you (*pointing to the bottom right*). Also imagine that the choice I'm about to invite you to make could determine the rest of your life, from that moment onward. Which of these two lives—the one on the left or the one on the right—would you choose?

Having asked thousands of people this question, we've noticed that they overwhelmingly vote for life number two. In all of our combined experience, less than a dozen have chosen life number one. In voting for life number two, people are choosing valued living over a life focused on controlling difficult thoughts, emotions, and other inner obstacles. This is what happens when you simply present the matrix point of view and invite clients to sort their experiences onto the matrix. Clients who, in all likelihood, came to see you to learn how to more effectively move away from or otherwise control unwanted inner experience instead readily choose to move toward what they care about. This both creates space and helps get them to start practicing psychological flexibility right away, given that they are choosing to move toward their values and making that choice in full view of some of the stuff that usually leads them to engage in away moves. In essence, the question heightens the contrast to the point that most people naturally choose appetitive control over aversive control.

Next, you can ask the fully fledged psychological flexibility question: "Are you interested in learning how to more easily choose to do this (*pointing to the upper right quadrant*), even in the presence of that (*pointing to the lower left quadrant*)?" Here again, in our experience most folks answer yes.

This seals the therapeutic contract because, once clients have answered these two questions, they have effectively signed up for psychological flexibility training as their overarching therapeutic objective. And in making that choice, they are already becoming more flexible. Now you and your clients have a yardstick with which to assess progress: Are they noticing that it's becoming easier to choose toward moves even in the presence of inner obstacles showing up?

Presenting the Present Moment as the Time to Learn

The work up to this point creates an ideal context for establishing that psychological flexibility (or whatever language you use to describe this, such as "the ability to choose to do what's important in the presence of inner obstacles") is a skill that can be learned, just like any skill. Then, because the mind has a way of telling us that we can learn something later, you might ask clients if they've noticed that learning can only take place in the present moment. Explain that because of this, the learning you'll engage in together will mostly take place in the moment.

When working with the matrix, the main skill that's practiced is noticing with the matrix. It's a bit like looking through a zoom lens. You can zoom both in time, from the scale of an entire life to that of a single moment, and in space, from the level of one person to a couple, a family, a group of people, or even an organization. The skill is primarily about looking through the point of view, not the content of what's seen. It's similar to developing a keen photographer's eye, which you accomplish by looking repeatedly through the lens of your camera at many different things until you start seeing what's important for you to see in order to take the pictures you want to take. Every look through the matrix provides practice in a skill that can be applied to any life situation, using whatever temporal and spatial resolution is best for the situation and the individual's goals. Note that the act of noticing itself is always taking place in the present moment, including noticing stuff that showed up in the past or noticing stuff we imagine showing up in the future.

Using the Therapeutic Relationship as the Context for Change

Some clients' difficulties are most salient in their interpersonal relationships. Further, difficulties in the way clients relate to others may stand in the way of doing effective work in session. With such clients, it can be useful to concentrate on interpersonal behaviors, using the therapeutic relationship as a training ground for noticing relating more effectively. As we'll explore in detail in chapter 7, the matrix is an effective tool for practicing therapeutic relationship–focused ACT (Schoendorff & Bolduc, 2014). The matrix can help clients notice the interpersonal functions of their behavior (in other words, their effect on others), and also help them shape and practice more adaptive interpersonal behaviors. The basic move is to show clients what shows up in your matrix in relation to what they do—provided you do this as a toward move—and to help them practice noticing the impacts they have on others.

Therapeutic relationship–focused work draws clients' attention to in-session behaviors that are the same as their problematic behaviors outside of session, along with improved in-session behaviors that could be effective outside of session. For example, a client who has trouble getting her needs met might not ask for what she needs from you. Perhaps she might always defer to you on setting the agenda, never sharing what she'd like to work on, or she may not ask if you offer sliding fees, despite facing financial challenges. In this case, you can draw her attention to this behavior when it shows up in session and encourage her to express her needs.

Informed Consent for Therapeutic Relationship–Focused Work

You can begin therapeutic relationship–focused work in the first session, which is why we are mentioning it now. However, note that this kind of work can be highly evocative for clients, so it's important to present a rationale for the work and obtain informed consent. You might present it along the following lines.

Therapist: Some people feel as though the stuff that shows up at the bottom left is like waves that they've been trying to either hold back or swim away from. Yet no matter what they do, eventually they can't hold them back, or no matter how fast they swim, the waves catch up with them. Then they get pulled under, tumble, and are swept out to sea. But there is an alternative: they could learn to surf. When you surf, you don't need to hold back the waves or run away from them, right? And not only are you not swept away, but you can even choose your direction. The thing is, it's possible that those waves may show up in here. They may be about our work, about us, or even about our relationship. This is actually normal and acceptable, and it will give us precious opportunities to notice those waves as they show up. Then you can learn to surf them toward the life and relationships you want.

Nudging Clients Toward Holding Themselves as Important

When clients list who is important to them, they often don't include themselves. When that happens, and especially if you intend to engage in therapeutic relationship–focused work, consider saying something like "I noticed that you didn't mention yourself as an important person to you," preferably mentioning this after they've listed their inner obstacles, as by then they can more easily notice whether inner obstacles have prevented them from naming themselves as important. Clients may say they just forgot, in which case they can be added to the list. Or they may respond with a story, perhaps about how they always put others ahead of themselves or about how difficult it is to see themselves as important. In the latter case, rather than get into the story, you can simply ask for permission to write "me" in the lower right quadrant of their matrix, perhaps saying something like "You're my client, and I notice that you are important to me." This may seem a bit invasive, yet if clients are unable to include themselves among the important people—most likely because of inner obstacles—this reminder that they are important, whether they see it or not, can be very effective in setting up an interpersonal context in which they really are at the center of the work. Besides, if clients are unable to hold themselves as important, it's unlikely that they can hold anyone else as truly important.

A General Note on Home Practice

As mentioned at the very beginning of this chapter, all matrix work is aimed at getting people to notice the matrix outside of session. Therefore, we continually invite people to notice their experience from the matrix point of view outside of session. Of course, that begins with noticing from the matrix point of view in session.

There is plenty of data indicating that clients who practice therapist-assigned exercises outside of session make the most progress. All cognitive behavioral therapy approaches thus assign homework to clients. And most therapists experience that clients may do the homework—or they may not. When they don't do the homework, this is often deemed a failure, by both therapist and client. And when clients fail, therapy will fail. With the matrix, although therapy is about maximizing opportunities to look from the matrix point of view outside of session, it is never about doing "homework." This isn't school, and we won't pass or fail clients. We simply invite them to explore noticing exercises. No exercise is compulsory. We only ask clients to commit to noticing: noticing if they do the noticing exercises and noticing if they don't. In either case, they will have succeeded in noticing, which is the fundamental exercise. For this reason, you will notice as you go through the steps that home practice exercises are systematically framed as noticing exercises.

Presenting home practice in this way ensures 100 percent compliance with practicing noticing outside of session. In addition, we've noticed that it makes it more likely that clients engage in noticing exercises, and that they do so of their own accord, rather than to conform and seek to appear to be a good client, known as *pliance*. Likewise, it makes it less likely that they'll resist doing the exercises because they don't want to be told what to do, known as *counterpliance*. Pliance and counterpliance, which we'll look at in more detail in chapter 2, can be major roadblocks to progress, so it's important to set things up so these dynamics are less likely to arise and easier to identify and work around when they do.

Furthermore, this approach (inviting clients to notice whether they engage in the exercises) promotes shaping the behavior of noticing. Clients vary widely in their initial ability to notice. As clinicians, we aim to shape noticing by starting wherever clients are in their abilities, rather than where we would like them to be. Initially, some clients may only be able to notice that they noticed after you prompt them at the beginning of the next session. This too counts as doing the noticing task, and clients can be reinforced for this success.

Noticing is hard and subtle work. At first, few of us are able to notice in real time, especially when we first start practicing noticing. Initially, most of us notice best as we look back to our past experience. That's okay. By practicing noticing, we gradually reduce the amount of time between our experience and behavior and noticing that experience and behavior. And eventually, we can begin to notice what might make a difference in the moment, or even anticipate what we might notice in the future. This is beneficial for everyone—clients and therapists alike. Therefore, we'll reiterate our recommendation from the introduction: that you engage in all the home practice exercises you invite your clients to do.

Step 1 Home Practice: Noticing Toward and Away Moves

Before wrapping up, invite clients to notice at least one toward move and one away move each day. Tell them they can either jot the toward and away moves they noticed on a piece of paper or write them on their matrix, which you'll send home with them. In any case, be sure to tell them that the exercise isn't about writing; it's about noticing. Also mention that if they forget to do this noticing, that's okay too. They will learn either way, as your sessions will be about practicing the noticing.

To prompt clients to practice this point of view, give them the matrix you worked on together and recommend that they keep it with them, perhaps carrying it in a pocket or purse—or on their phone if you worked on a whiteboard and can photograph the result. Another great way to promote matrix practice is to suggest that clients present the matrix point of view to others.

How to Notice and Flexibly Sidestep Potential Traps

Using the matrix in clinical practice is about using flexibility to train flexibility. Just because we outline one way of doing things is no guarantee that the work will go smoothly and according to plan. Everyone is different, and some clients may respond in ways that trip you up. Sometimes you may get in your own way. We know we do. This section outlines some of the potential traps and sticky points we've encountered in our training and clinical practice and offers guidance on how to deal with them and keep the work flowing.

Explaining vs. Pointing

You may find yourself trying to "explain" the matrix point of view. However, using the matrix is more a matter of pointing toward experience than about explaining the matrix. It's like a finger pointing at the moon—the moon of the client's experience. There's no need to explain the moon, especially given that each of us can only access our own experience. Just keep pointing at the client's experience until you notice the client noticing it. Some clients may start looking in the distance before responding, others may pause or smile, and yet others may shift their pace, tone, or posture somewhat. Any of these can be outward signs that clients are noticing their experience. The more you pay attention to how it looks when clients are noticing the moon of their experience, the more you'll come to recognize the signs of individual clients' noticing. And because you don't have access to clients' direct experience, noticing these signs will provide you with much better guidance to orient your work than debating with them about the content of experiences that only they can see.

For this reason, as you use the matrix diagram with clients, we encourage you to point at the different quadrants of the matrix as much as possible and to also invite your clients to point at the matrix. You might notice that this helps cut through words and stuck stories—that it helps clients notice their experience from the perspective of their experience, rather than through the obscuring filter of their stuck stories. Remember, the main goal is noticing, and when clients notice this experience, they are standing in the perspective-taking zone that lies beyond stuck stories.

Sorting for Clients Rather Than Getting Clients to Sort

You may find yourself sorting clients' experience into the matrix. For example, after a client has explained what brought her to you in some detail, you may be tempted to use the matrix to show her how her story can be seen through the point of view of the matrix. This may work, but given that the goal of matrix work is to get clients to sort their own experience through the matrix, the sooner you get them doing it, the better.

An effective way to get clients started on sorting is to volunteer some of your own experience and engage in sorting it in front of them. When working with individuals we usually don't give examples of who or what is important to us, leaving the field open for clients to freely choose who or what is important to them. However, sharing some of your inner obstacles and away moves can prime the pump and help them notice and share their own challenges. This can also be a highly validating move, since clients might notice that the two of you share some common obstacles and away moves. Just be sure to share low-intensity examples so you don't risk putting your own suffering and difficulties at center stage.

Think of sorting with the matrix as a peg-in-the-hole game, and let clients put the pegs in whatever holes they choose. Their own experience will show them what shape of peg goes into what shape of hole. Verbal instructions and rules are less useful than gentle encouragement to play the game. Further, because individuals are really the only ones who can see the shape of their experience, telling clients what should go where might not be fitting or helpful. Nothing guarantees that the way their experience appears to you is the way it appears to them. Indeed, if you push them too hard to sort in a particular way, what they will experience is your pushing, and then they'll start sorting more in relation to that than to their experience. This would defeat the purpose of the game.

You may have heard the saying "Tell me and I forget. Teach me and I may remember. Involve me and I learn." The matrix takes that saying to heart and, from the outset, involves people in the learning process. We invite clients to notice their experiencing, especially the feelings, thoughts, and urges that show up throughout the day.

Trying to Get Clients to Sort Correctly

Clients may initially sort in ways that seem wrong to you. For example, they may put "not feeling anxious" in the lower right quadrant (what is important), sort external obstacles, such as "an irate boss," in the lower left quadrant (inner obstacles), and, quite commonly, describe thoughts, feelings, and other inner experiences—things that couldn't be seen on a video camera—as away or toward moves. That's okay. Let them sort "incorrectly." As they become more adept at sorting with the matrix, they'll gradually sort in ways that are more effective and workable.

If you can't picture something a client says she does as a toward or an away move, you can do something we call "shaking the bag." For example, if a client says one of her away moves is avoiding, say something like "Yes, and when you avoid, what is it that you can be seen doing?" Notice that this question points toward behavior. After you've shaken the bag in this way, the client may offer a clear description of an observable behavior—or not. If not, especially early in matrix work, it's best to write what the client says, word for word, than to continue shaking the bag, which is likely to make the client feel she's failed at answering your questions. As a result she may be less inclined to continue playing the sorting game with you.

Trying to Sort It All

The point of presenting the matrix is not to get a highly detailed picture of everything clients may notice in all the quadrants of the matrix. The point is to get them to successfully look through the point of view, as if taking a photograph and describing some of what they see in each of the four quadrants. Again, you want clients to win at this sorting game. An effective way to help ensure that is to reinforce whatever they're able to do and then move on.

Frequently Asked Questions

Do I have to present the matrix in the order presented in this chapter?

You don't necessarily have to start at the bottom right and finish at the top right. After you learn how to connect client experiences to the matrix diagram, you can adjust the sequence if that seems called for. That said, we have noticed that the sequence we've presented works well. It begins with who or what is important (reflecting values, which lie at the beating heart of ACT), and it concludes with what clients can do to move toward their values (or committed action, which is vital to making ACT work).

The first question you ask is important because it primes the person's responses for the session. It's like a fork in the road. One path, the "toward fork," heads toward talking about values. The other, the "away fork," usually heads toward talking about problems and being stuck. If you start on the left, you may predispose your clients to talk about problems and seek fixes for them. Then, later, when you want to talk about values and how to go about moving toward them, they may have a harder time of moving to the right-hand side of the matrix.

While starting on the right-hand side is generally best, there are more options for where to go next. For example, after inviting clients to name who or what is important, you can ask them what they could be seen doing to move toward who or what is important, completing the right side before moving to the left. That said, we recommend that you first practice the sequence outlined in this chapter. Once you're adept with this approach, you can cover the quadrants in any sequence that seems workable.

What if clients say nobody or nothing is important to them?

We used to first ask, "What is important to you?" Every so often, a client would respond, "I don't know," "nothing," or "nothing anymore." Since we switched to starting with the question "Who is important?" we haven't had a single client answer "nobody." However, should a client answer "nobody and nothing," here's what we used to say to great effect: "Imagine you could choose between two lives, one in which someone or something was important and one in which nothing was important. Which of these two lives would you choose?" In all likelihood, clients will say they'd choose a life with important people and things. Then you can simply write, "Someone or something important" in the lower right quadrant and say something along these lines: "Let's make helping you identify who or what is important to you part of our work, okay?"

What if clients come looking for solutions?

Many of our trainees fear that presenting the matrix so early in therapy might spook clients, especially those who come seeking solutions. We've found that clients are generally quite receptive to the matrix in the first session—provided that the therapist takes the time to connect to their experience of what brings them to therapy, reflects it back to them, and then asks for permission to present this point of view. You can usually seal the deal by getting them to choose between the two potential lives and answer the psychological flexibility question outlined above ("Are you interested in learning how to more easily choose to move toward who or what is important, even in the presence of inner obstacles?").

Of course, some clients may still press for solutions—for example, by asking, "Yes, but how do I do that?" You can answer along the following lines.

Therapist: The good news is, this is a skill you can learn, and we'll work on that. In fact, and this may sound weird, you've already practiced it some by choosing to move toward what matters while in the presence of your doubts and questions about how to do that and all the inner obstacles you've noted in the bottom left. Between now and the next time we meet, see if you can notice some of your toward and away moves, and maybe even some of the inner stuff that shows up around those moves.

Also, bear in mind that the matrix is a tool to help people find their own solutions by identifying what works for them. There aren't many ready-made solutions for human life problems. What works always depends on the context. If we give clients ready-made, generic solutions, they likely won't be a good fit, and clients may never be able to fully embrace them. Or they may work, but only for a short while. Giving clients a tool for identifying and testing their own solutions—the matrix—is much more likely to have a lasting impact on their ability to live a valued life.

Going Deeper

In this first glimpse of what goes on beneath the hood in matrix work, we'll discuss priming, connecting clients to their experience and to the matrix, sidestepping stuck stories, and holding ideas lightly. We'll also discuss some of the relational framing processes that may play a role in the step outlined in this chapter.

Priming

No matter how you approach introducing the matrix to clients, you'll be talking with them about moving toward who or what is important to them in the presence of unwanted inner experience. Yet as discussed in the preceding FAQ section, most clients arrive expecting to tell you about unwanted stuff, such as depression, and how to get rid of it. During step 1, you introduce them to a different perspective, priming them to look at things from a new point of view.

So let's take a deeper look at priming. As you read the word "apple," you're almost instantly primed so that you can respond more quickly to the word "orange." Hundreds of experiments have shown the effects of priming. One famously primed some students by having them do a task that included a lot of words associated with the elderly (Bargh,

Chen, & Burrows, 1996). Then those students and a control group were asked to walk down a hallway, and those who had been primed with words related to the elderly walked down the hallway more slowly. Priming happens automatically and is unavoidable, explaining why first impressions are so important—and why we encourage you to introduce the right (toward) side of the matrix first.

Taking a step back, the popular media primes people to come to therapy looking for solutions to problems. If you start by asking about their problems, you're priming them to expect a solution. This is especially the case among clients seeing clinicians who can write prescriptions.

Working with the ACT matrix is a process, not a cut-and-dried solution. In fact, a big part of the process is helping people notice that spending a lot of time looking for solutions to problems might be part of their problem. Through the matrix, they can shift focus and see that it may be more beneficial to instead engage in an ongoing, daily process of discovering behaviors (both internal and external) that promote valued living. Attachment to fixing problems often gets in the way of that process.

Ultimately, given that people are already primed to seek solutions to problems, if you start by presenting the left (away) side of the matrix, clients can fall into long stories about their problems and thwarted solutions. Then you'll face the task of interrupting a well-rehearsed story, which can be tricky.

Connecting Clients to Their Experience and to the Matrix

In matrix work, the clinician's task is to show clients the matrix point of view so that they can start sorting their own experience through it. A big reason this is so effective is that the matrix sets up a functional contextual point of view. The vertical line represents the context (both inner and outer) and the horizontal line represents the function of behavior (toward or away). Functional contextualism and the matrix offer a useful point of view for deriving and choosing new behaviors that promote valued living.

Given that the matrix represents common and fundamental human experiences like sensing, thinking, feeling, and doing, it's a relatively simple task to relate clients' experience—and your own experience—to the matrix diagram. However, for most people it's a new way of looking at living, and as with anything new, using it takes some practice. There are many ways to connect clients' experience with the matrix and help them get used to looking at their world through this point of view, and new ways are being derived every day. Once you become fluent in these skills, you may derive your own matrix approaches. If you do, be sure to let us know!

Sidestepping Stuck Stories

Clients show up with stuck stories. That is to be expected, and therapists would be very surprised if they didn't. Furthermore, clients typically want to use the therapeutic context to tell their stuck stories. But the thing about stuck stories is that they tend to get therapists stuck as well as clients. If it's a really good, juicy story about sex, deceit, and intrigue, the therapist may get drawn into the story and end up stuck there too.

Plus, if these stories get clients stuck outside of session, they will also get them stuck in session. One reason is because stuck stories tend to lead to sticky questions that just keep everyone stuck. Again, it's natural for clients to ask sticky questions, in large part because they're usually looking for straightforward solutions to complex problems. Part of them knows the solution won't be straightforward, but that won't keep them from asking questions like "So what do you think I should do the next time this happens?"

Can you feel the stickiness of that question? You are being asked to provide a specific course of action for the client to take in a context in the future, when neither you nor your client can know the exact nature of that future context. If you do, you may be setting yourself up to later hear, "I tried doing what you told me to do, and it didn't work."

You need to elegantly and deftly sidestep those questions before allowing them to fall onto the matrix. So in this case, you might answer, "You just said the words 'What do you think I should say the next time this happens?' Where would saying those words go on the matrix?"

In this way, you simply invite the client to sort. This skill is central to matrix work and is at the heart of verbal aikido, which we'll describe in detail in chapter 4. We mention it here because you're probably already hearing these kinds of stuck questions from clients. The matrix offers you a new way of responding to them.

Here's another example. Imagine a client says, "You're saying I should practice this matrix all the time? I'm not good at remembering to practice anything." Notice the feelings that show up inside of you as the client says "all the time." If you're like most therapists, "all the time" feels stuck, and that's usually the function of these words when clients send them your way. The word "should" feels pretty stuck too, right? And "I'm not good at remembering to..." encapsulates an entire other story of stuckness. Once you have a bit of practice with the matrix, you'll choose to sidestep questions like this because they are so obviously sticky. The best tactic may be to first take the time to validate what your client is experiencing, then simply invite her to sort the statement onto her matrix.

When you notice stuck stories that clients send your way, also notice that these stories are part of the process that keeps them stuck. This is just what people do when they're unable to look at their experience from the psychological flexibility point of view.

Holding Ideas Lightly

You might notice that the presentation we recommend includes statements like "It's a point of view that some people have found useful." Notice that such statements don't make any wild promises about this point of view. Nor do we suggest that this point of view should always be used. We're simply demonstrating a point of view. In ACT, this is referred to as holding ideas lightly, and it's part of the essence of psychological flexibility. If we were to hold the matrix point of view tightly, we might become rigid and not notice when another point of view might be useful.

So as you work with clients, model holding ideas lightly. For example, you might use the words "show up." Here's an example: "So you noticed your friend walk into the room, and you noticed that your friend was frowning. When you saw that frown, what showed up inside you? What did your mind tell you it meant?" This stands in contrast to inquiring from a mechanistic, cause-and-effect point of view: "So you saw your friend walk in the room wearing a frown. How did that make you feel?" The latter suggests a causal link between the frown and your client's feelings—a relationship that doesn't necessarily exist—and therefore constitutes a rigid and inflexible use of language. There can be a whole range of responses to seeing a friend with a frown, and which response shows up depends on a lot of factors. The next time the client sees her friend frowning, she might have a completely different response. Clearly, the friend and the frown don't make the client feel any particular way. That's why we use wordings like "shows up" a lot. Inviting clients to notice what shows up is a more flexible use of language and invites a more flexible response.

In the Frame

According to relational frame theory, we frame ourselves into being. While this may sound strange, consider this: When you arrived in the world, you didn't know yourself as "me." You were just a tiny being doing stuff largely in response to your sensory experiences. As you acquired language, you gradually learned to verbally differentiate yourself (me-here) from others (you-there). Soon the "me" took on all kinds of meaning for you as you built a story about "me."

When we show people the matrix to ease them into the psychological flexibility point of view, we train them to extend that view of self by having them purposely notice the self going through the process of living on at least two experiential dimensions: experiencing the world and the self in terms of five-senses and inner experiencing, and experiencing them in terms of the purpose of their behaviors (toward and away). When working with the matrix, we regularly return to these two basic discrimination tasks because they work so well to expand the way clients actively frame their experiences and their sense of self as the moments of their lives unfold.

As the matrix is introduced in step 1, the most useful framing behaviors you teach clients to engage in involve the discrimination of hierarchical and deictic relations. In RFT, frames of perspective are known as *deictic frames*. They include here-there, now-then, and me-you. Developing the ability to notice these three differences in perspective leads us to become self-reflectively aware of ourselves. These three frames are key to a stable sense of self and perspective-taking skills, and they are also involved in empathy, compassion, and flexibility. At any moment in time, our sense of self is a collection of myriad experiences and our framing of those experiences. "I feel good now," "I felt angry yesterday," "I am going to the store," "I went to the store," "I failed the exam," "I got a raise," "I hugged my partner," "I want to get better," "I feel hopeless," "I'm depressed," "I will get better," "I'll only get worse," "I'm a fighter," "I'm a loser"—all such statements are parts of the constellation that constitutes our sense of self at any given time. When healthy, this sense of self remains flexible and open to new framing and experiences. When the emphasis is on the products of the framing, such as feeling a particular way (as it often is in typical interactions and our inner discourse), this may lead to inflexible framing of self-experience and inflexible self concepts. By activating deictic and hierarchical framing, using the matrix can expand and broaden our sense of self to include all of our experiences as normal parts of life and lead to broader definitions of what we may accomplish. In other words, it gives us a broader sense of who we are and who we could be.

Hierarchical framing involves framing something as being a part of something else (A is an attribute or member of B). Activating deictic framing can also activate hierarchical frames in the sense that all inner experience and behavior are framed as part of one's experience and one's self. The result of this process of learning a framing repertoire is the emergence of a stable perspective and sense of self, sometimes called the observing self. This process, which is central to ACT, is best thought of as a behavior that provides us with a perspective from which to notice all of our experiences and choose our behavior.

When people sort with the matrix, they are, de facto, in the position of I-here-now, looking at their experience as if it were someone else's: you-there-then. This often allows them to gain enough distance and perspective to choose behavior in line with their values. This type of process may even be central to all framing. Perhaps it emerges from seeing ourselves in others' eyes. Before you can frame something as "the same," "different," "opposite," "more than" or "less than" something else, and so on, you first have to step back and take perspective on the things framed by these relations. So at heart, the matrix is about deictic and hierarchical framing, and adopting the matrix point of view exercises the observing-self muscle.

As you'll see throughout this book, using the matrix activates a complex network of relations to help people derive new relations and choose valued action even from within the most stuck situations. Depending on client history, some of these frames may start activating from the get-go, moving things along. For example, when clients sort behavior into toward and away, they may start to perceive away moves as less attractive if they frame them as standing in opposition to toward moves. Similarly, they may start to perceive toward moves as more attractive if they frame them as part of moving toward something or someone important to them. Both of these new frames could increase the probability of toward moves and thereby contribute to greater flexibility in a given situation.

Step 1 Checklist

Use this checklist (available for download at http://www.newharbinger.com /33605) to guide your practice of the strategies outlined in this chapter.

What I did

- [ ] I asked for permission before setting the agenda and presenting the point of view.

- [ ] I took time to connect with and reflect my client's experience of what brought her to therapy.

- [ ] I invited my client to sort her experience, as stated in her own words, into the matrix.

- [ ] I asked "Who is important?" before "What is important?"

- [ ] I framed toward moves as toward who or what is important, and away moves as away from inner obstacles.

- [ ] I asked my client who chooses who or what is important and who can notice who or what is important, inner obstacles, and whether what she does is a toward move or an away move.

- [ ] I invited my client to choose between a life mostly about away moves and one mostly about toward moves.

- [ ] I asked the psychological flexibility question, framing it as the skill of more easily choosing toward moves in the presence of inner obstacles.

- [ ] I made it clear that the work is about practicing a present-moment skill.

- [ ] I invited my client to engage in a daily practice of noticing toward and away moves.

- [ ] I made clear that she need not necessarily do daily practice; that all she has to do is notice if she does it and if she doesn't.

- [ ] I shared some of my matrix in a way that didn't put me at center stage.

What I didn't overdo

- [ ] Explaining

- [ ] Sorting for my client

- [ ] Letting my client proceed with telling a stuck story

CHAPTER 2

Step 2: Understanding the Effectiveness of Away Moves

In step 1 we focused on presenting the entire point of view to clients without focusing on any particular side or quadrant of the matrix. One of the strengths of the matrix is precisely that it allows people to look at the whole picture all the time, increasing the chances that all the ACT processes will be recruited to help clients move toward a valued life. In this chapter, we'll look at an effective and experiential way to get clients to notice how their away moves are working and whether these away moves are workable or keeping them stuck. We think of this step as constituting a broad functional analysis of away moves. It also provides an opportunity to validate how easily clients can get stuck and clears the way for them to engage in a different way of looking for a solution to their difficulties.

Looking at Away Moves from the Workability Point of View

In this second step, which can generally be accomplished in a single session, you'll establish workability as the main criterion for valued living. The aims of this step are threefold: validating clients' experience, exploring the long-term unworkability of stuck loops, and reorienting clients' attention to the impact of stuck loops on valued living. In effect, this trains clients in a values-centered functional analysis of away moves. In our experience, clinicians and clients respond well to this phase.

Functional contextualism is, at root, a pragmatic approach. Its truth criterion is workability, meaning what works to get people where they want to go. Workability is a contextual criterion in that it can only be evaluated for a particular situation and in light of a statement of goals or values. From a functional contextual point of view, nothing is inherently true or false; actions or statements are simply workable, or not, only inasmuch as they prove effective in helping people move toward their goals and values.

A functional contextual perspective is ideally suited to interventions and clinical practice because it sidesteps the potential traps of trying to assess the "truth" (or otherwise) of thoughts—a place where clients and clinicians often get stuck. Instead, the emphasis is on the workability of behavior under the control of those thoughts and other inner experiences.

Settling-In Noticing Exercise

We generally begin the second session, and all subsequent sessions, with a short noticing exercise. It helps clients tune in to what's showing up for them as they start the session and also invites them to identify or choose what they'd like to work toward in this session.

ACT is commonly seen as a mindfulness-based treatment. Mindfulness has been defined by Jon Kabat-Zinn as "paying attention in a particular way: on purpose, in the present moment, and nonjudgmentally" (1994, p. 4). The heart of matrix work is promoting a particular way of noticing (another term for paying attention), the purpose of which is to promote valued living. In some ways, it's a more specific way of noticing than in most formal mindfulness training approaches, while still being fully compatible with those approaches.

One interesting aspect of using the matrix is that the particular kind of mindfulness it trains can be developed without engaging in formal mindfulness exercises, making it useful to a broader range of clients. And although we typically use the matrix without teaching any formal mindfulness exercises, we do like to use the following short noticing exercise, which can help both clients and therapists settle into the room and into the session.

> As a way to start this session, I'd like to suggest we do a short settling-in exercise. Then, if it feels useful to you, we could start our future sessions with it.
>
> Take some time to let your body find a comfortable position in your seat. You're looking for a position comfortable enough that you won't have to move around over the few short minutes this exercise takes.
>
> Once you've found a comfortable position, see if you can let your gaze rest in front of you. Then, if it's comfortable for you, let your eyes close gently, or just keep them open. Now let your attention come to rest on your breathing, just noticing the movements in your chest and belly, as you inhale…and as you exhale…
>
> If you notice your attention wandering away from the breath, that's perfectly normal. See if you can just note where your attention went and then gently bring it back to noticing the movement of your breath in your chest and belly…
>
> Now see if you can turn your attention toward the thoughts and feelings you've had about today's session, either since you got up this morning or over the past couple of days. See if you can simply notice whatever shows up…
>
> Now see if you can identify or choose who or what is important to you for today's session. Again, see if you can simply notice whatever shows up…
>
> Now, if you're willing, see if you can form the intention to take steps, in this session, to move toward who or what is important to you for today's work…

For my part, I'll support you as best I can in taking those steps…

Now bring your attention back to the room, back to the chair on which you're sitting, back to the two of us here to work together today… And when you feel ready, if you've had your eyes closed, let them open again.

Debriefing this exercise provides a great opportunity to reinforce noticing. When debriefing, reinforce any and all noticing nonjudgmentally—without getting sucked into the content of what clients say they noticed. Responses along the lines of "You noticed that. Well noticed" can be quite effective. Then, when after this first debriefing you put the important items that showed up for your client on the session agenda, this further reinforces your client for identifying what's important.

As therapy unfolds, you can adapt this exercise to reflect where your client is in the process. In some ways, this brief exercise encompasses a large part of what the matrix trains: noticing sensory experience in the moment, noticing thoughts and emotions that show up, identifying or choosing what's important in the situation, and forming an intention to move toward who or what is important. Further, it allows you, the clinician, to state your intention to support your client's toward moves as best you can, and it establishes the therapeutic relationship as a context in which toward moves can be explored and reinforced.

We've also found that the invitation to notice when attention wanders away from the breath, and to gently turn back to noticing the movement of the breath in the body, is a potent metaphor. It speaks to noticing when we wander away from moving toward who or what is important and then gently returning to the choice to behave like the person we want to be. This is the key to valued living: noticing when our actions have drifted away from who or what is important and gently turning back to valued action.

In fact, this settling-in exercise can help anyone prepare for any important task or encounter in life. Through it, we connect with our bodies; notice the thoughts and emotions that have shown up when anticipating the event; identify or choose what's important to us in the situation; form an intention to take steps to move toward what's important; and establish an intention to support ourselves as best we can in taking those steps. So perhaps you'll want to practice a short induction along these lines before clinical sessions and other meaningful professional and personal situations for a week or so. You may start noticing interesting differences.

Once you've debriefed the settling-in exercise, you can move to debriefing the broader noticing exercise offered as home practice for step 1.

Home Practice Debrief

To debrief the step 1 home practice, simply ask clients what they've noticed since the previous session. Did they notice that they noticed at least one toward move and one away move each day? Did they notice that they didn't notice?

As you engage in this debriefing, remember that you're trying to shape your clients' noticing behavior. Behavior is shaped by starting with whatever clients are presently doing—their current repertoire—and then reinforcing successive approximations of the target behavior, in this case noticing and, more broadly, demonstrating psychological flexibility. When debriefing home practice exercises, the target behavior is noticing with the matrix from the perspective of the client's own experience. Seek to reinforce any approximation of this kind of noticing.

Clients will have noticed either that they noticed toward and away moves or that they didn't. In either case, they've succeeded in their home practice because they noticed. If they notice that they didn't notice any toward or away moves, you can ask them if, looking back, they are now able to notice a few toward or away moves over the past week. Most clients can, allowing you to reinforce this later, in-session noticing. Remember that noticing in real time is an advanced skill; at first, most of us only notice when we look back on our experience. And that's okay.

Gradually, and with practice, the time lag between behavior and noticing decreases, and eventually people are able to notice in the moment—at times primed by anticipating what they may notice ahead of time. Depending on the context, these different forms of noticing—in the past, in the present, or anticipating noticing ahead of time—may be more or less useful, and more or less easy. Throughout the client's journey with noticing, remember that as a clinician your goal is not for clients to comply with your requests; it is for clients to learn to notice their own experience through the matrix point of view.

Functional Analysis of Away Moves

The matrix can be a highly effective tool for assessing the effectiveness of away moves and helping clients notice how these moves can keep them trapped in stuck loops. At this point in step 2, we offer a step-by-step exercise that allows clients to notice the workability of their away moves from three perspectives: how effective away moves are in reducing unwanted inner content in the short term, how effective away moves are in reducing unwanted inner content in the long term, and how effective away moves are in helping them move toward who or what is important.

For this exercise, it's best to use the client's filled-in matrix from step 1. Clients may have added some toward and away moves that they noticed during their home practice since the previous session. If you filled in the matrix on a whiteboard rather than on a piece of paper, consult the photo you took so you can use those away moves as you proceed with the present exercise.

Assessing the Short-Term Effectiveness of Away Moves

As you'll recall, when we explained how to fill in the matrix in chapter 1, we suggested you leave about one inch of space to the left of the vertical line, and about half an inch to the right. Draw two vertical lines in the upper left quadrant to divide that space into two columns, and draw one vertical line in the upper right quadrant to create one column. (Figure 4 shows these columns.)

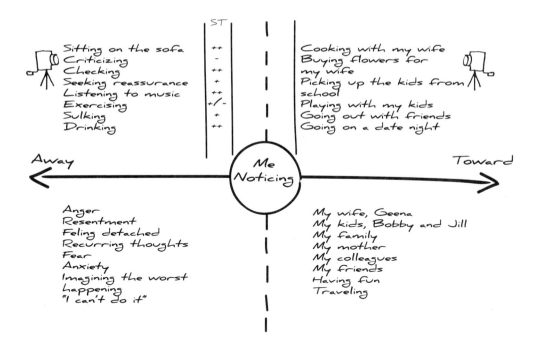

Figure 4.

Next, write the heading "ST," for "short-term," at the top of the leftmost column. Then invite clients to rate the short-term effectiveness of their away moves—clarifying that, for this exercise, "short-term" can mean anything from a few milliseconds to days, weeks, months, and in some cases even years—and give a few examples, perhaps along the following lines.

Therapist: Sometimes when I feel angry, I can raise my voice and leave. At first it brings me great relief. Yet it barely takes a second before I start feeling guilty, ashamed, and possibly even more angry. In fact, if I blinked I might miss noticing that bursting out is effective in the very short term, given how quickly I then feel worse. On the other hand, say I avoided an uncomfortable family Thanksgiving dinner. This might be effective for a number of months, until next year's invitation comes along. So it's only effective short term too because, in the long run, it isn't effective. So something that's effective in the short term can be effective for barely seconds or for quite a while before the effect wears off.

Next, ask clients to assess their experience of the short-term effectiveness of each of their away moves using the following scale of pluses and minuses: +++ means highly effective; ++ means quite effective; + means somewhat effective; 0 means no effect; – means makes it somewhat worse;– – means makes it significantly worse; and – – – means makes it much worse.

You may need to redirect clients to keep them on track with the rating system. Minds are great at creating stories, and as discussed in chapter 1, clients usually come in with stuck stories. They can easily get diverted by offering explanations or reasons for their away moves, rather than simply rating their effectiveness. This is likely to derail the process. To prevent this from happening, it's helpful to start by offering that for now you're only going to look at ratings, rather than explanations, and that later there will be plenty of time to look at things in more detail and consider possible explanations. Assuming clients agree to this, you can then gently direct them back to assigning ratings any time they start giving you explanations.

Sometimes clients notice that their away moves have different effects in different contexts. This is excellent, because it reflects more nuanced noticing. In such cases, you can simply note two ratings separated by a slash, as is done for "Exercising" in figure 4.

Finally, and importantly, be sure to orient clients to their own experience. Explain that these ratings aren't about how they think an away move ought to work, but about how well they've noticed that it works. It can be useful to say you don't have any preconceived notions about it, and more useful still to demonstrate this by showing that you aren't attached to any preconceived ratings based on how you think a given away move ought to work. Figure 4 provides an example of how a client might apply the rating system.

Most clients notice that their away moves are effective in the short term. This provides a perfect opportunity to validate that their away moves make sense. After all, they work. This allows you to model perspective taking, as you're looking at the situation from the client's perspective. Here's a dialogue illustrating how that might play out.

Therapist: So most of the things you do to move away from what you don't want to feel or think work. They're not stupid; they make sense. They work.

Client: Well, yeah, in the short term…

Therapist: Yes, in the short term. In a minute, we'll look at how effective they are in the long term. For now, I'm noticing that, from the point of view of your own experience, they do work. The fact that our away moves work could go a long way toward explaining why we keep on doing them—especially when it's the only way we know of for dealing with this stuff in the lower left.

We can't overemphasize how important it is to invite clients to notice their own experience when assigning these ratings, as in all matrix work. The more they sort their own experience, the more effective the intervention will be. One potential trap is trying to get clients to say what you expect them to say. A bigger trap is to say it to them, perhaps in the form of psychoeducation, telling them how their away moves work or don't work before they've had a chance to evaluate them in light of their own experience.

Occasionally, clients rate most of their away moves as ineffective. From the perspective of learning theory, they're most likely unaware of the reinforcing contingencies at play. That doesn't matter. The aim here is to shape the behavior of noticing their own experience, not to get them to give answers congruent with learning theory. So if clients, based on their present noticing repertoire, notice that their away moves make things worse in the short term, you can reinforce them for noticing and move on. When we take that approach, we notice that clients not infrequently return to these initial evaluations, either later in the session or in future sessions, and share that they now notice how their away moves are effective in the short term. That said, arriving at this realization isn't essential to effective matrix work. If clients can't notice that their away moves are at least somewhat effective in the short term, it's best to just move on.

Next, read back the client's responses: which away moves are effective in the short term, which have no effect, and which make things worse. As we've suggested, you'll be most effective if you don't show obvious bias in favor of responses indicating that away moves are effective in the short term.

Assessing the Long-Term Effectiveness of Away Moves

Next, write the heading "LT," for "long-term," at the top of the second column in the upper left quadrant, then invite the client to assess the long-term effectiveness of his away moves. Simply put, away moves are only effective in the long term if the unwanted stuff has never come back, or if it's become less intense, less frequent, or somehow less important. Again, keep the dialogue focused on ratings, not explanations. You could say something along the following lines.

Therapist: Now let's look at the long-term effectiveness of your away moves, rating them with a similar scale. See if you can notice whether, since you've been doing this particular away move, the stuff you don't want to think or feel has become smaller, less intense, or less frequent. If so, then rate it with pluses, using three pluses if it's never come back. If you've noticed that the stuff in in the lower left has actually grown more intense, more frequent, more troublesome, or more important, then rate it with minuses.

Most clients notice that even if their away moves are effective in the short term, they are often ineffective in the long term, and oftentimes have made things worse. Figure 5 illustrates these typical responses.

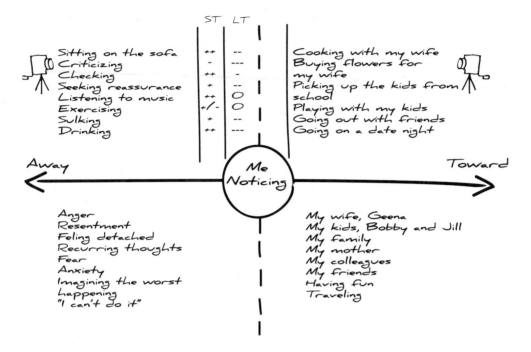

Figure 5.

As with ratings for short-term effectiveness, clients aren't always accurate in tracking the long-term effectiveness of their away moves. A few may even rate all of their away moves as effective in the long term. In such cases, you can gently prod using questions such as "You've rated this away move as quite effective, with two pluses. Have you noticed that since you've been doing this away move, your anxiety has become less important in your life and diminished a fair amount, say two-thirds?"

Then again, if clients stick with their ratings, just roll with it. There could be many reasons for their ratings. They may be hooked by their mind telling them that certain away moves ought to work. Their experience may be that some of their away moves feel milder than the stuff in the lower left quadrant, such as full-blown fear. Another possibility is that they're reacting against a perception or assumption that you expect them to conform to a rule that their away moves must be ineffective. Lastly, there is the possibility that these away moves are indeed effective, in which case they may actually be workable behavior—provided they don't stand in the way of moving toward who or what is important. As in most situations with the matrix, it's best to reinforce clients for noticing, whatever form that noticing takes in the moment.

Next, read back the client's responses: which away moves have no long-term effect, which make things worse, and which, if any, are effective in the long term. Here again, you'll likely be most effective if you don't show obvious bias in favor of responses indicating that away moves make things much worse. You don't need to put your finger on the scale to get clients to renounce their away moves. In fact, away moves are perfectly understandable. In situations where it feels like the house is on fire, away moves beckon as brightly as emergency exit signs. There's nothing wrong with going for the emergency exit, and in some situations doing so makes a lot of sense. It's just that this rarely takes us where we want to go. In fact, emergency exits often lead to dark, narrow, and dirty alleyways.

Uncovering Stuck Loops

Once clients have rated the short-term and long-term effectiveness of their away moves, the picture that typically emerges is that away moves work in the short term but tend to have no effect or make things worse in the long term. You can then say, "So your away moves work… And they don't work." After a short pause, you might add, "That's how all of us can get into stuck loops." With most clients, this elicits a flash of recognition.

You can then draw a stuck loop directly on the client's matrix (see figure 6). It's a spiral that starts out in the bottom left quadrant ("So this stuff shows up"), curves leftward to the upper left quadrant ("And you do some of this to move away, right?"), then spirals back down ("And it comes back, doesn't it?") and back up ("And you do more of this?"), and continues spiraling inward ("And on and on?") until there's no space left. Then say, "If you do this again and again, you get stuck. And when you get stuck, life can lose vitality and meaning." This often constitutes an "aha moment" in therapy.

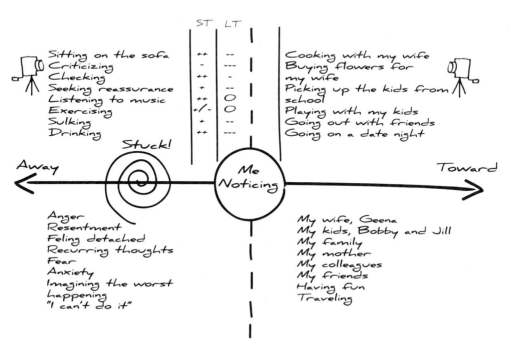

Figure 6.

Because stuck loops involve repeatedly engaging in away moves, they often cause clients to experience hopelessness and harsh self-judgments. Noticing particular stuck loops and naming them can therefore be a powerful intervention, opening the door to change. Help clients see all aspects of their stuck loops, including the fact that stuck loops have their uses and are often good for something. This validates clients' experience and helps them take in the broader consequences of engaging in these behaviors. Once a loop is identified, invite clients to describe it using their first name; for example, "This is Tom stuck in his 'turning down invitations and watching movies' loop."

Assessing the Effectiveness of Away Moves in Terms of Who or What Is Important

After uncovering and validating clients' stuck loops, invite them to consider their away moves from a third perspective: in terms of their effectiveness in moving toward who or what is important to them in life. This reinforces how central workability is for valued living.

Moving to the right-hand side of the matrix, write the heading "I," for "important," at the top of the column to the right of the vertical line. Then set forth the following seven-point scale, which differs slightly from that for short-term and long-term effectiveness in moving away from unwanted inner content: +++ means an away move is very effective for moving toward who or what is important; ++ means it's quite effective; + means it's somewhat effective; 0 means it moves the client neither toward nor away from who or what is important; − means it moves the client somewhat away from who or what is important; − − means it moves the client a good distance away; and − − − means it moves the client a great distance from who or what is important. (You can see a filled-in example in figure 7, which we provide at the end of this section.)

As you proceed, once again keep the discussion focused on ratings, rather than explanations. In many cases, clients notice that their away moves also move them away from who or what is important. However, this isn't always the case. Some away moves may help them move toward who or what is important. A common example is exercising. People may engage in exercise as a way to move away from stress, and they often notice that this is effective in the short term but less so in the long term. However, they may still notice that it helps them move toward health, which may be important to them.

Once the client has rated all his away moves in this column, run through each of the ratings, then wrap up this exercise by simply going over his ratings in all three columns.

You can also revisit any stuck loops that were uncovered. Clients commonly notice that away moves are effective in the short term, not so effective in the long term, and rarely a reliable way to move clients toward who or what is important. And even when they function to help move toward who or what is important, this is generally done at the cost of vitality. However, and as always, the key is to connect with clients' experience, rather than trying to prescribe anything or force them to adopt preconceived notions.

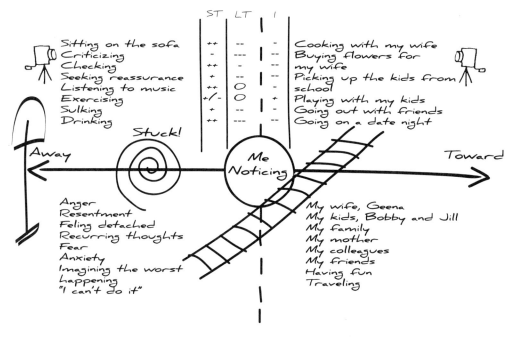

Figure 7.

When Away Moves Are Also Toward Moves

As the preceding exercise reveals, sometimes away moves are effective in moving people toward someone or something important to them. This leads to an interesting situation wherein it isn't necessary to change the behavior itself; rather, the functions of that behavior are targeted for change. Through therapeutic work, behavior that was previously under the aversive control of unwanted inner stuff (away moves) can gradually come under the appetitive control of values (toward moves). This is where the power of derived relational responding, which promotes the transformation of functions, comes into its own.

For an illustration of this dynamic at work, consider the clinical case of a sixty-year-old client who had lived with obsessive-compulsive disorder (OCD) for over five decades (Schoendorff, Purcell-Lalonde, & O'Connor, 2013). His main obsessions involved recurring images of his daughters being tortured. He also had a profound sense of not being good enough at whatever activity he engaged in and felt that he didn't deserve any of the breaks he got.

When working with the matrix, he listed his main away moves as going jogging (which he did at least twice a day), calling his daughters, calling other people, doing volunteer work, doing crossword puzzles, avoiding (by which he meant that he had stopped teaching), and doing "other things," such as cooking. All of these were effective in the short term, but in the long term none of them made any difference to the intensity or frequency of his obsessions and anxiety, so he gave them all a long-term rating of 0. However, all of his away moves, with the exception of avoiding, were also effective in helping him move toward who or what was important to him.

It turned out that his compulsive behaviors were potentially steps toward valued living. However, for them to become that, he needed to engage in them under appetitive control rather than as moves away from his obsessions and anxiety. Through the three-column functional analysis outlined above, he noticed that his away moves, which he initially viewed as entirely problematic, could also be toward moves. Gradually, by simply noticing when he engaged in them as away moves and when as toward moves, he noticed that he was increasingly engaging in them as toward moves. By the end of therapy he was free of compulsions, despite still engaging in the same behaviors. His only overt behavior change was returning to part-time teaching.

The same repertoire of behaviors that had once been under rigid aversive control had, through the power of noticing through the matrix point of view, come under appetitive control and thus been transformed. For example, even though the behavior of regularly calling his daughters looked the same, he noticed that it felt different to call them to connect with them and be a part of their lives, rather than to check whether they were still alive. He also noticed that his relationship with his daughters was improving and deepening.

Wrapping-Up Metaphor: Man in the Hole

One effective way to wrap up this session is with the classic Man in the Hole ACT metaphor (Hayes, Strosahl, & Wilson, 1999). You can even draw elements of the metaphor on clients' matrix diagram, lending it extra visual strength. Here's a dialogue that illustrates how presenting this metaphor in the context of the matrix might play out.

Therapist: Imagine that when you start out in life, they blindfolded you and gave you a bag to carry on your back. You didn't know what was in the bag, and you couldn't see that you were standing in a field full of holes. So you started walking along. You walked in a straight line, then you walked toward the right, then you walked toward the left. And one day you fell into a hole. Still blindfolded, you started groping in the bag, where you found a shovel. Hole, shovel… You started digging. Who wouldn't? (*At this point, you can draw a shovel pointing up on the left-hand side of the matrix, with the blade in the away moves.*) You tried digging steps with this away move (*naming the first away move*). You tried digging tunnels with this away move (*naming the second away move*). You tried digging ramps with this other away move (*naming the third away move*). You tried digging with all of these other away moves (*listing the remaining away moves*). But since you've started digging, have you noticed the hole getting any smaller?

Client: No, it's been getting bigger!

Therapist:	Right. Maybe a shovel isn't the most effective tool for getting out of holes? What would be a better tool?
Client:	Maybe a rope?
Therapist:	A rope might work, but I'm no good at drawing ropes. And besides, you'd need someone to hold the other end or anchor it. What else?
Client:	A ladder?
Therapist:	Right, a ladder! As it happens, I'm a purveyor of pretty good ladders. But there are a couple of problems. First is the fact that, since all you've ever used is this shovel, you might understandably be holding on to it for dear life. So what's the first thing to do if you want to grab hold of the ladder?
Client:	Drop the shovel.
Therapist:	Yes, though that's easier said than done! Have you ever held tightly onto a stick? Do you recall how it felt when you finally let go? Do you want to try with this pen here? *(Client grabs the pen.)* Okay, now hold on to it as tightly as you can with both hands for about thirty seconds. *(Pauses.)* And now release it and notice the sensations in your fingers.
Client:	They're stiff. It's uncomfortable.
Therapist:	Exactly. As you let go of the shovel, you may experience some discomfort or even temporary pain. But that's not all. If the only thing you've ever tried is digging, even if you let go of the shovel and grab the ladder, chances are you'll try to use the ladder for…
Client:	…digging.
Therapist:	Right. And then your mind will tell you, "This isn't…"
Client:	"…working!"
Therapist:	Exactly, and your mind will be right, because ladders don't work for digging.

At this point, you can draw a ladder going from bottom left to upper right, as illustrated in figure 7. To conclude, point out that continuing to dig is just human nature. You can reflect that people, yourself included, commonly do this, even when they notice that their away moves mostly work in the short term, often make things worse in the long run, and don't reliably move them toward who or what is important in life. Here's one possible presentation.

| Therapist: | Sometimes people come to see me hoping I have a power shovel, with massive horsepower and a microprocessor-controlled platinum-diamond |

blade. The bad news is I don't. And it's also good news, because if I did, it would only make your hole bigger. All I have is a basic shovel, just like yours, and I sometimes find myself digging in my own hole. In our next session, we'll look under the hood at what it is that makes us keep on digging even when we notice that it's not workable.

Step 2 Home Practice: Noticing the Workability of Away Moves

Noticing toward and away moves remains part of the home practice after this second step, and for all six steps, as this is the primary skill we're training in clients. If clients connect with identifying stuck loops, encourage them to notice stuck loops and pay closer attention to their away moves, particularly their short-term and long-term effectiveness and how workable they are for moving toward who or what is important. If clients seemed to resonate with the Man in the Hole metaphor, you can cast away moves as digging and encourage them to notice the effectiveness of digging and whether it works to move them toward who or what is important. Be sure to tell clients that they need not do anything different at this stage other than simply notice their toward and away moves in the normal course of their day.

How to Notice and Flexibly Sidestep Potential Traps

Remember, using the matrix in clinical practice is about using flexibility to train flexibility. To that end, in the following sections we outline some potential traps that are especially likely to arise in step 2 and offer effective strategies for flexibly sidestepping them.

Speaking for Clients

The goal of matrix work is to help clients notice their own experience from the perspective of their own experience. To promote this, adopt a style of interaction characterized by asking clients about their experience rather than telling them about it. Make frequent use of questions such as "What do you notice when you look at that aspect of your experience?" Of course, this isn't just about the wording of the questions; it's equally about your tone and attitude. Regardless of what your mind may say in the moment, bringing genuine curiosity to the task of gently pointing to different aspects of clients' experience works best.

Letting sentences linger unfinished, thereby giving clients a chance to complete them, also works well. An example would be wrapping up discussion of the short-term effectiveness column with something like "So your away moves aren't stupid. They work…" This gives clients an opportunity to complete the sentence with something like "yes, in the short term." Remember that you're seeking to reinforce every instance of clients' noticing, even if your mind tells you that their noticing is off track or somehow wrong.

Similarly, when you present a long metaphor, such as the Man in the Hole, try to get clients highly involved, asking them questions and playfully letting the conversation take unexpected turns as they engage with the metaphor. Think of it as taking clients sightseeing in a part of town they're unfamiliar with. Along the way, you point at buildings, landmarks, people on the street, and so on, and ask them what they see and how they see it. If your commentary is too intense and pointed, it can stand in the way of clients noticing for themselves.

Gradually, as clients get better at noticing their experience, they'll start noticing in ways that work for them.

Seeing Behavior on the Left-Hand Side as Exclusively Away Moves

Although the main behavioral discrimination of the matrix is between actions to move toward who or what is important and actions to move away from unwanted inner stuff, it's important to remain flexible about how clients connect with this discrimination.

Although it is rare, clients sometimes sort behaviors that seem to be on the left side as toward moves. For example, we once had a client who initially sorted his pot smoking as a move toward a desirable feeling rather than a move away from unwanted inner experience. Rather than insisting that his pot smoking had to be an away move, we validated that he noticed it as a move toward a particular feeling. When it came to assessing the effectiveness of that move, we just invited him to notice how effective pot smoking was to move toward that feeling in the short term and in the long term, and how effective it was in helping him move toward who or what was important to him.

We don't claim that the matrix point of view can capture all the possible contingencies surrounding all possible human behavior, much less that it provides a conceptual description of behavior. Rather, it is a simple point of view that captures enough common experience that everybody can connect it to their own experience and easily sort both their experience and their behavior from that perspective. One way to reflect that is to refer to away moves as "away or under the control of the stuff at the bottom left."

As for that pot-smoking client, in the next session, unprompted, he volunteered that he'd taken a second look at his pot smoking and noticed that it also served to help him move away from a kind of tension he felt inside. The fact that we went along with how he initially noticed it (as a toward move rather than an away move) probably created the space for that noticing—not that it would have made much difference if he'd continued to notice pot smoking as a move toward a desirable feeling.

Overly Pathologizing Subclinical Clients

When using the matrix in some contexts, such as in coaching or with organizations, and more generally with subclinical clients, it may be better to present stuck loops as potential traps rather than trying to force folks to admit that they're stuck when they may not feel they are. In these contexts, you may not have to engage in a detailed exploration of the effectiveness of away moves, and the Man in the Hole metaphor may not be especially useful. A brief presentation of stuck loops may work better. Such a presentation would consist more of psychoeducation than of experiential exploration. In such cases, you can integrate step 2 right after your initial presentation of the matrix by drawing the loop once you've simply asked if the stuff in the bottom left ever came back after an away move, and continuing this for a few cycles as you draw a stuck spiral. Alternatively, you can briefly address this before presenting hooks, as outlined in chapter 3, where you'll find pointers about presenting stuck loops differently. The important point is to titrate the exploration of stuckness to match how stuck a given client feels.

Frequently Asked Questions

What if clients say their away moves are working?

As discussed, some clients may have trouble noticing the effectiveness or ineffectiveness of their away moves. In such cases, simply go along with whatever clients are noticing in the moment and invite them to keep noticing over the next week. Likewise, when using the Man in the Hole metaphor, sometimes clients say that letting go of the shovel is a relief and brings on nice sensations, even after we've invited them to do the experiential exercise of tightly gripping a pen for thirty seconds. Don't insist that there's temporary discomfort or pain associated with releasing; simply validate whatever the client notices.

What if clients say a behavior is effective in the short term and the long term, and also works for moving toward who or what is important?

This question sometimes comes up in our training workshops, though we've never seen a client notice this. That said, if a client rates a behavior as effective in all three dimensions, perhaps it simply isn't a problem behavior; in fact, it could be part of a workable solution. If you doubt this is the case, remember that the point is to reinforce noticing, not obtain "correct" answers. For the time being, simply say that this particular away move seems to be highly effective in the short term and long term, and as a toward move.

What if clients say they must dig steps, tunnels, or ramps?

In our presentation of the Man in the Hole metaphor, you might have noticed that we linked client away moves to common forms of trying to get out of holes with shovels, such as digging steps, tunnels, or ramps. If you do this, clients probably won't offer different forms of digging as ways to get out of the hole.

Going Deeper

In this chapter, we'll go deeper by discussing pliance and counterpliance, and then turn to why it is so essential to keep the focus on clients' experience and to broaden the scope of their noticing of that experience. Then, as is our wont, we'll conclude with a discussion of various forms of relational framing that may be activated in step 2 and the types of transformation of functions this step aims for.

Pliance and Tracking

Two of the biggest obstacles people face in noticing their matrix from the perspective of their own experience are pliance and counterpliance. As mentioned briefly in chapter 1, pliance is complying with a rule given either by others or by one's own mind. In practice it looks like one is following the rule pretty much for the sake of following the rule, although the rule is actually followed because, in the past, doing so resulted in social reinforcement from significant others. In pliance, coordination between the behavior and the rule results in reinforcement. This leads people to respond to their experience not from the perspective of the whole of their experience (as when noticing the full matrix point of view), but from the narrow perspective of what they imagine other people—or their minds—expect of them. For its part, counterpliance is disobeying a rule given either by others or by one's own mind. In practice it looks as though one is disobeying the rule pretty much for the sake of disobeying the rule, although the rule is actually disobeyed because gaining the disapproval of a particular person or group has in the past resulted in reinforcement.

Children typically follow rules pliantly early in their developmental history. As a small child, you probably put on your coat in winter because your mom, your dad, or another caregiver told you to. And in all likelihood you were reinforced—at first possibly through enthusiastic approval—by whomever proffered the "put on your coat" rule. That was pliance. Early in life, pliance generally isn't a problem; it's just how we learn to follow the rules that can often be helpful as we navigate life.

Returning to our example, over time you might have begun to notice that putting on your coat in winter not only pleased your parents, but also kept your body warm and comfortable. This is *tracking*—noticing the broader consequences of following a rule, beyond simply receiving approval, or not receiving disapproval, from the rule giver.

In normal development, before or around the time when tracking behavior emerges, children tend to respond in a counterpliant manner. You may recall times when you didn't put on your coat precisely because you were told to. In counterpliance, as in pliance, the individual's interaction is with following the rule itself, rather than with the broader consequences of following or not following the rule. Both pliance and counterpliance can lead to inflexibility because they narrow people's awareness of consequences to whether a rule is followed or defied, insulating them from noticing broader consequences that might better and more flexibly guide their behavior. That said, responding in pliant or counterpliant ways can at times be workable.

Pliance and counterpliance are not developmental phases that we grow out of. In certain contexts, most of us will behave in either pliant or counterpliant ways. This is often true of clients in the therapy context, perhaps especially in regard to homework. Given that school is often a context in which pliance and counterpliance are broadly reinforced, it's fairly common for clients to react to home practice exercises as they would to school homework. Taking care not to call home practice exercises "homework," as recommended in chapter 1, can only go so far in preventing that.

When clients don't do the home practice, or when they do it but you perceive a forced quality in how they report on their home practice, you may want to gently alert them to what might be going on. You might initiate a conversation about whether they perhaps felt guilty for not having noticed or whether they felt compelled to do the home practice. This can set the stage for later orienting them to the pitfalls of responding to what they imagine you expect of them. To get a feel for how you might do this, consider the following dialogue with Joshua, who came back after his first session saying he hadn't done his "homework," as he called it.

Therapist: So what you're saying is that you noticed you didn't notice toward or away moves. You know what? That's noticing right there.

Client: Yes, but I feel bad that I didn't do it. It's been a crazy week.

Therapist: It sounds like you had a hard week. Are you maybe feeling like you're back at school and haven't done your homework, and the teacher's going to be mad at you?

Client: (Laughs.) Well, almost…

Therapist: I guess we can't stop your mind from doing that to you, but this isn't school. There is no homework—only exercises that you can explore. They're mostly about noticing. And the cool thing about noticing is that we can do it anytime. For example, I could ask you right now to see if you can now notice a couple of toward and away moves you did over the past week. Maybe you can't, and that's okay too, because you're noticing that you can't.

Let's say Joshua then reels off a few toward and away moves he engaged in at work and at home. After complimenting Joshua for noticing those, the therapist then concludes as follows.

Therapist: You know, doing or not doing the exercise can be a toward move, an away move, or a bit of both. The thing is, the only person who can notice whether it's a toward move or an away move—or both—when you do something or don't do it, is you. At first, noticing this can be hard and confusing, especially if you've been accustomed to doing or not doing things because of what you thought people or your mind expected you to do. But you'll soon get the hang of it. And when you do, you may notice that you start doing and not doing things because you choose to.

As a flexible matrix practitioner, be on the lookout for possible pliant and counter-pliant behavior. Moments when clients are able to notice that they're responding in pliant or counterpliant ways offer ideal opportunities to orient them toward tracking their own experience and thereby increase their flexibility in noticing. When doing that, it's best to use everyday language, perhaps asking whether they've noticed that they're doing something because you suggested doing it (or whether they're feeling resistant to doing something because you suggested it). Of course, getting them to pliantly acknowledge their pliance, or counterpliantly deny their counterpliance, won't be helpful. If you feel that something like this may be happening, it's best to move on. We'll get back to this important issue in chapter 5.

Broadening Clients' Awareness of Their Experience

In order to promote broad derivation of functions (and to reduce any tendency toward unworkable pliance and counterpliance), it's important to create verbal contexts that help clients connect as directly as possible with their experience, rather than with their thoughts about what you expect from them. They've probably already heard from either others or their own minds that their behavior isn't working, so continuing to connect with thoughts about their experience, rather than their experience itself, is likely to result in more of the same.

If you succeed in helping clients connect with their experience, they'll typically be in contact with a broader range of stimuli than just their thoughts or whatever part of their experience they tend to focus on: emotions, bodily sensations, five-senses experience, or dwelling in the past or future. This broadening will multiply the ways in which they frame their behavior and help them derive new functions—in this case, aversive functions for away moves and appetitive functions for toward moves. For this reason, it's best to use questions that invite noticing and to reinforce all signs of noticing, no matter how imperfect they may seem, rather than trying to get clients to answer in a certain way.

When clients notice that their away moves are effective in the short term, it's likely that they're connecting with their experience and thereby deriving broader functions. They probably notice coherence between their behavior and its function. In the absence of this broader perspective, it's all too easy for clients to not notice the effectiveness or functions of their away moves. Many underlying processes can lead to this kind of inflexibility. Perhaps a client generally attends to mental events such as self-blame and is therefore so critical of his avoidance that he can't see that it provides an effective escape from fear. Alternatively, a client may feel that others don't understand him—a view you're likely to reinforce if you don't take the time to connect with his broader experience; for example, by observing that substance use is often a highly effective short-term strategy for changing one's inner experience.

In the Frame

We'll begin our discussion of the types of relational framing at play in step 2 with a brief foray into basic behavioral processes, particularly reinforcement. We take this tack because people often get stuck due to the short-term reinforcing functions of their away moves. In case it's helpful, bear in mind that there are two types of reinforcement: *positive reinforcement*, in which the future probability of a behavior is increased when something is added to the environment (generally something appetitive), and *negative reinforcement*, in which the future probability of behavior is increased when something is removed from the environment (generally something aversive).

Because away moves allow us to escape or avoid aversive stimuli (largely difficult thoughts or uncomfortable feelings), they can seem very attractive. Indeed, they have a short-term appetitive function (when anxiety is rampant, exiting the situation seems most attractive), even if these functions are themselves largely under aversive control in that they serve to move us away from an unpleasant experience (negative reinforcement). In some cases, such as the pot-smoking client mentioned earlier in this chapter, reinforcement may come from adding a feeling that was previously absent (positive reinforcement).

From a functional contextual perspective, whether a given form of reinforcement is negative or positive is no more set than whether a given behavior is an away move or a toward move. A behavior noticed as a move away from something could just as well be noticed as a move toward something else. So for the behavior of smoking pot, it's possible to see negative reinforcement due to subtraction of a stimulus, say a sense of emptiness, from the context. However, it could just as well be seen as positive reinforcement due to the addition of another stimulus, say a pleasant buzz. Given that positive and negative reinforcement are just ways of seeing behavior, from a functional contextual perspective the "right" way of seeing is the one that works best to help move you and your client in the direction you want to move.

When we present the matrix, we generally explore a dynamic of moving away from unwanted inner experience versus moving toward who or what is important because this captures most people's experience. Looking primarily at moves toward and away from values is less likely to connect to people's experience. In our clinical experience, clients don't engage in behavior to move away from values. Plus, an initial focus on whether their behavior moves them away from values tends to put people into a more evaluative frame of mind. We've found that it's more effective to first connect with most people's experience, and everybody has experienced moving away from unwanted inner stuff and moving toward someone or something important.

Furthermore, the matrix targets behavior under the aversive control of inner experience because when we are controlled by aversive functions (such as extreme fear of being scrutinized by others), our behavioral repertoire narrows (seeking the nearest exit). In the process, our sensitivity to broader elements of the context (such as the meeting we wanted to attend and the important people we wanted to meet) vanishes, as does our ability to distinguish between our five-senses experience of the moment (other people are in the room) and what our minds are telling us about it (it's so awful that we can't stand another minute of it). In technical terms, when aversive control reigns, behavior is less responsive to changes in context and psychological flexibility withers.

Among the goals of conducting a functional analysis of away moves is to provide a context for clients to derive stronger appetitive functions with respect to toward moves than are available for moving away from unwanted inner experience, and to promote the derivation of aversive functions to their away moves. If fleeing via the nearest exit spits you out in a dark alley where you're still beset by anxiety, exit signs might appear somewhat less attractive. With this in mind, we'll now turn to how various relational frames can be used to derive new functions for away moves.

Assessing the short-term and long-term effectiveness of away moves is an instance of temporal framing. Generally, the long-term temporal frame will prompt the away moves to derive aversive functions because they are mostly ineffective. In those cases where away moves are effective long-term, they may derive some additional appetitive functions, which is okay. Perhaps these away moves represent effective control strategies, though they aren't necessarily workable unless they're also effective for moving toward who or what is important.

When we assess away moves in terms of their effectiveness in moving toward who or what is important, we frame them in terms of hierarchy (behavior that is part of one's values) and temporality (in which behavior promotes moving toward values over time). This gives rise to a relational frame–based definition of values: behavior that is part of one's values and an ongoing pattern that, over time, is effective for moving toward values.

Values carry highly appetitive functions, so when away moves and values lie within a frame of opposition—in other words, when away moves take the place of potential toward moves—aversive functions are derived for these away moves. However, evaluating away moves in terms of whether they are effective in moving toward who or what is important is best used to frame the work more broadly and as a gentle invitation to look at the workability of away moves as part of a life that is largely about moving toward. This is because simply noticing that away moves can move us away from values can in itself be aversive. Therefore, it's important not to overuse that kind of framing, as it may make the framing itself, and the person who offers it, aversive. In other words, the client will soon want to move away from looking through these frames, and maybe even from you, and thus get into another stuck loop.

On the other hand, framing away moves in terms of their effectiveness in moving toward who or what is important is highly recommended when those behaviors actually can serve to move the client toward who or what is important. In such cases, behavior under the aversive control of unwanted inner experience, which is generally life narrowing, can gradually move under appetitive control to bring increased vitality. As discussed earlier in this chapter, when away moves are effective for moving toward values (as can be the case for exercising), these away moves can gradually derive broader appetitive functions. This increases the probability that clients will come to engage in them as toward moves: behavior under the appetitive control of what is important. And that's the stuff a valued life is made of.

Ultimately, in terms of relational framing, everything we do is aimed at helping clients frame their situation more flexibly. In other words, we help clients engage in flexible framing of events and experiences that had been framed inflexibly. It's impossible to predict with 100 percent certainty what will help them do that. The best we can do is try to create conditions that increase the probability that they'll begin to frame their experience more flexibly, without inflexibly trying to force this new, more flexible way of framing on them.

Step 2 Checklist

Use this checklist (available for download at http://www.newharbinger.com /33605) to guide your practice of the strategies outlined in this chapter.

What I did

- [ ] I debriefed the home practice in a flexible way.

- [ ] I offered that we could look at the client's away moves a bit more closely.

- [ ] I invited my client to first look at the short-term effectiveness of his away moves in terms of moving away from unwanted inner experience.

- [ ] I validated that away moves can be effective in the short term and conveyed that my client's away moves make sense and aren't stupid.

- [ ] I invited my client to look at the long-term effectiveness of his away moves in terms of moving away from unwanted inner experience.

- [ ] I helped my client identify and name at least one of his stuck loops.

- [ ] If my client's ratings allowed for it, I validated that away moves both work (in the short term) and don't work (in the long term).

- [ ] I invited my client to look at the effectiveness of his away moves in terms of moving toward who or what is important to him.

- [ ] I validated whatever my client noticed regarding the effectiveness of his away moves in terms of moving toward who or what is important.

- [ ] Throughout the exercise, I was able to gently reorient my client toward rating effectiveness rather than giving explanations.

- [ ] I used the Man in the Hole metaphor, presenting the metaphor in an interactive way and involving my client in the dialogue.

- [ ] As a home practice exercise, I invited my client to continue noticing his toward and away moves, paying particular attention to noticing the effectiveness of his away moves in the short term, in the long term, and for moving toward who or what matters.

What I didn't overdo

- [ ] Trying to force my client to say his away moves are effective in the short term, ineffective in the long term, or ineffective for moving toward who or what is important

- [ ] Letting my client give lots of explanations and veer off track

CHAPTER 3

Step 3: Hooks and the Problem with Control Efforts

Human beings have developed amazing abilities to control their environment. We control it so well that we can live in some of the most hostile environments on Earth— and even in outer space. We have our finely honed individual and collective intelligence to thank for this. And because we are so accustomed to controlling the environment around us, it's only natural that we would seek to control our inner environment: thoughts, emotions, memories, mental images, and the like. However, the inner world isn't so amenable to such control, and in many cases inner-directed control efforts don't work. In fact, efforts to control our inner experience are often the root cause of getting stuck.

The natural pull to control inner experience in the same way that we control the outer world of five-senses experience is made all the stronger when we have difficulties noticing the difference between the two worlds. When we don't make that discrimination, we naturally tend to interact with thoughts, emotions, and other inner experiences as if they were among the things out in the world of five senses that we can control.

Step 3 is about looking under the hood at what makes us seek to control inner experience. It consists of two parts. The first part is an experiential exploration of the sharp contrast between our ability to control the world of five-senses experience and our inability to control the world of inner experience. The second part helps clients identify which inner experiences can get them stuck through an extended presentation of the Hooks metaphor, accompanied by a worksheet.

Home Practice Debrief

Before debriefing the step 2 home practice, you might open this session with the short settling-in exercise from the beginning of chapter 2. Afterward, debrief the exercise by reinforcing any and all noticing, for example, by saying, "You noticed that? Well noticed!"

Next, turn to the previous week's home practice. Ask clients whether they noticed toward and away moves over the past week. If they did notice away moves, did they also notice the effectiveness of those moves, in terms of both short-term and long-term effectiveness in controlling unwanted inner experience, and in terms of working to move them toward who or what is important? If appropriate, refer to stuck loops or invoke the Man in the Hole metaphor and refer to the away moves as digging.

A Brief History of Human Control

After debriefing the home practice, remind clients that at the close of the previous session you promised to look "under the hood" to see what keeps us stuck in away moves, even when we notice that those moves are largely ineffective or make things worse in the long term, and that they rarely move us reliably toward who or what is important. We recommend beginning by offering a brief historical overview of the development of human control skills. The following dialogue illustrates how you might do this.

Therapist: We humans are unique in our ability to control the world of five-senses experience. We can control the temperature in our homes through heating and air-conditioning systems and our body temperature through clothing. We can communicate across long distances and even into space, travel at incredible speed, and successfully fend off many deadly creatures, whether predators or microscopic pathogens. What makes this possible? Is it that we have sturdier bodies, stronger muscles, sharper claws or teeth, or more powerful jaws than other animals?

Client: No, it's because of our brains.

Therapist: Right. It's the stuff between our ears that has allowed us to control the world of five-senses experience like no other living species. Consider the progress we've made in our ability to control the world outside the skin over the past two to three thousand years, since the times of the ancient Greeks and Romans. Yes, they had houses, and some of the very rich even had primitive central heating systems, but they had no glass in their windows and no air-conditioning.

They had clothes, of course, but not the technical clothing of today. They primarily traveled by foot, on horseback, or in fairly rudimentary carts or ships. For telecommunications, they had to go up a hill with a piece of polished metal and hope for sunshine so the person on the next hill could catch the reflection. Now we can teleconference with anyone via the Internet. Medicine was a touch and go business, with doctors as likely to kill people as save them. You get my drift. And all of this progress in a short two to three thousand years is thanks to our minds.

When humans encountered things in the world of five-senses experience that they didn't like or wanted to change, they gave it some serious thought and maybe bounced ideas off each other to come up with solutions. As a result, we've made great strides in controlling many unwanted aspects of our external experience. But what about the world of inner experience—the world of our thoughts and emotions? How much progress would you say we've made since the days of ancient Rome?

Client: Not much...

Therapist: Not much at all. Isn't there something strange there?

A Side Note on the Evolution of Cognitive Control Technology

Consider the following statement that spells out the essence of the most advanced technology for controlling thoughts and emotions—cognitive therapy: "If you are distressed by anything external, the pain is not due to the thing itself but to your own estimate of it; and this you have the power to revoke at any moment" (Aurelius, 1964, p. 120). This quote isn't from a cutting-edge psychology text, but an extract from the writings of Roman emperor Marcus Aurelius, penned sometime in the second century AD. Oddly, it does a pretty good job of summing up a central principle of cognitive therapy: that we can reduce our distress by changing our evaluations of our inner experience. Doesn't it seem a little strange that our most advanced technology for controlling thoughts and emotions hasn't progressed much beyond a principle stated almost two thousand years ago? Imagine if our most advanced modes of transportation relied upon the same technological principles that prevailed in Marcus Aurelius's time.

To be clear, we don't think the trouble lies with cognitive therapy per se. We feel it comes from trying to apply control to a realm where it isn't appropriate.

An Experiential Exploration of the Futility of Control in the Inner World

Now that you've set up a context applying a frame of comparison to the human ability to control the world of five-senses experience and the world of inner experience, it's a perfect time to experientially explore important differences between these two worlds. The dialogue that follows, which makes use of the metaphor of a lie detector, illustrates how you might do this.

Therapist: How about we look a bit more closely at how things work in the world of thoughts and emotions?

Step 3: Hooks and the Problem with Control Efforts   67

Client:	Okay.
Therapist:	Let's look at thoughts first. How many times have you thought of a purple unicorn over the past week?
Client:	Zero.
Therapist:	Great, so what I'm going to ask you to do should be easy. Here it is: No matter what you do over the next thirty seconds, don't think of a purple unicorn or anything that makes you think of a purple unicorn. This isn't about proving anything to me; just see if you can just notice your inner experience. If you notice anything that makes you think of a purple unicorn, just wave your hand so I can see it. I'll do the same, so we both get to look stupid.
Client:	Okay. (*Falls silent and almost immediately starts waving her hand, as does the therapist.*)
Therapist:	Okay, I think twenty seconds is long enough. What did you notice?
Client:	Unicorns everywhere!
Therapist:	Isn't that strange? You hadn't thought of a unicorn for the past week. Yet all I have to do is tell you not to think of one, and suddenly unicorns are everywhere!
Client:	(*Chuckles.*)
Therapist:	Now consider this piece of paper. If we wanted to get rid of it, what could we do?
Client:	You could throw it in the trash can.
Therapist:	Right. And knowing my two-year-old, he might just fish it out. So that would be effective in the short term, but maybe not the long term. What else?
Client:	Burn it.
Therapist:	Yes! Burning it would work. Would it ever come back?
Client:	No.
Therapist:	So in the world of five-senses experience, if there's something we don't like, we can think about it and come up with a way to get rid of it. It might take a couple of attempts, but we can do it. Not so in the world of thoughts, right? Yet see if it's not the case that your mind regularly tells you not to think of something or to think of something else instead. What are the chances you can do that?

Client:	No chance.
Therapist:	Right. So now let's consider whether it's the same for emotions. Do you know about lie detectors?
Client:	Yes.
Therapist:	Then you probably know that it's a lie to call them lie detectors. What they react to are changes in skin conductance and blood pressure that arise due to anxiety and stress. So now imagine that the FBI, CIA, NSA, Department of Homeland Security, and a few other agencies, the names of which are so secret that if I told you I'd have to kill you, have developed the most sensitive stress and anxiety detector ever. This thing can detect the tiniest signs of stress and anxiety. Now imagine that we put you in the most comfortable chair and wire you to this device. Your job is to not feel the slightest bit of anxiety and stress. Given how comfortable the chair is, that shouldn't be too hard.
	Oh, by the way, the chair is on a platform, sitting right on top of an automated trapdoor wired to the machine. If you experience even the slightest stress, the trap door will open. And just to give you even more motivation to not feel any anxiety and stress, we've put the platform above a pool of sharks that haven't been fed for weeks. How long do you suppose you'd remain in that comfortable chair?
Client:	(Chuckles.) Not long. Five seconds maybe...
Therapist:	Wow! I'm not sure I'd last that long! At any rate, see if it's not the case that your mind regularly insists that you shouldn't feel something but should feel something else instead. Has your mind ever told you that you should not, on any account, feel any stress or anxiety? (Points fingers to head like a gun.) That this time it's vital! What chance have you got?
Client:	No chance.
Therapist:	Hmm... But maybe it's different for positive emotions? Let's see. If you can make yourself feel the most joy you've ever felt in the next twenty seconds, I'll give you a million dollars. Let me start the clock... Go!
Client:	(Remains silent.)
Therapist:	Okay, twenty seconds gone. What did you notice?
Client:	I couldn't feel it.
Therapist:	Right. And even so, how often does your mind tell you, "Don't think this; think that!" or "Whatever you do, don't feel this!" or even "Why don't you feel this!"?

Client:	(Chuckles.) Pretty much every day.
Therapist:	Weird, no? Yet it kind of makes sense that our minds do this. They've been so successful in helping us find ways to control the world of five-senses experience that it's only natural that when they turn to the world of inner experience, they would suggest more control. But as we've seen from these experiments, this doesn't seem to work in the world of inner experience.
Client:	No. It actually looks like it makes things worse.

The Rules of Outer vs. Inner Control

The preceding dialogue illustrates how you can guide clients through an exploration of the huge difference in our ability to control inner versus outer experience—from the perspective of their own experience. This puts you in a good position to invite clients to notice that these two worlds seem to operate according to different rules.

Therapist:	It appears that there are different rules for the world of five-senses experience and the world of inner experience. In the world of five-senses experience, the rule goes something like this: "If you don't like it, think about it long and hard, try different things, and eventually you can get rid of it or control it." For the world of inner experience, the rule seems to be "The more you try to get rid of it or control it, the more you're stuck with it!" Maybe that's part of how we get stuck—by trying to apply the rule for the world of five-senses experience to the world of inner experience.

Sorting Five-Senses and Inner Experience

Next, you might tell clients that, given these two different rules—pertaining to the world of the five senses and pertaining to the world of inner experience—it can be useful to practice noticing the difference between five-senses and inner experience. Then again, because this discrimination is central to matrix work, just sorting with the matrix often suffices to allow clients to notice the difference. If it looks as though a client readily discriminates between five-senses and mental or inner experience, you don't need to invite her to specifically practice noticing this difference.

If you do want to train this important difference directly, you can give clients two index cards and invite them to label one "5-S," for five senses, and the other one "M/I," for mental or inner experience. Prepare similar cards for yourself, then say something along the following lines.

Therapist:	For the next sixty seconds, let's practice noticing the difference between five-senses experience and mental or inner experience. Take one card in

each hand. Then see if you can notice where your attention goes. When you do, raise the hand with the card that best corresponds to your experience of the moment.

It's a bit like sorting cards from two different decks, red-backed and blue-backed, that have been shuffled together, except the cards are your moment-to-moment experience. The red-backed cards would be anything you perceive through one or more of your five senses: sight, hearing, smell, taste, or touch, such as the feel of your clothes on your skin. The blue-backed cards would be everything else: thoughts, emotions, images, memories, or inner bodily sensations, like rumblings in your belly or discomfort in your chest—basically anything that doesn't come in through one of your five senses. And just so you don't worry about looking stupid doing this, I'll join you and sort my moment-to-moment experience with these cards too.

We have found it helpful to say something along the following lines to warn clients about some common traps they may encounter when doing this exercise.

Therapist: This isn't about sorting perfectly; it's about sorting. It also isn't about sorting your experience of even just one second ago; it's about sorting your experience in the present moment, no matter what your mind tells you about how you've just sorted it—right or wrong. When doing this exercise, people often experience confusion or notice thoughts such as "This is stupid," "What's the point of this?" "I don't know what kind of an experience this is," "I'm not noticing any particular experience right now," or "How can this possibly help me with my problem?" (specifying the client's presenting problem). Well, what kind of experiences are those?

Client: Mental!

Therapist: Right, mental. Basically, mental or inner experience includes anything that doesn't come through one of the five senses.

When debriefing this exercise, simply reinforce all noticing, taking care not to seem to reinforce one outcome over another, such as five-senses experience over mental or inner experience. As the client shares, you can gently ask whether what she's sharing is inner or five-senses experience, if that seems helpful or appropriate. You can also share some of your own experience of the exercise—which you may notice will change from one instance of doing the exercise to the next. As ever, when sharing your experience, do it from a position of equality and authenticity, without getting hooked by the thought that you should share some of your experiences over others in the service of teaching clients some predetermined lesson.

We sometimes recommend that clients practice this exercise for a minute or so each day. A number of clients have reported this exercise really helped them get less entangled in their thoughts, clearing the way for valued action. Clients can practice with or without the cards. If practicing with the cards, they may want to find a quiet, private place to do so. They can also practice while showering, cooking, walking down the street, or even driving—without the cards, of course.

Interestingly, in a currently ongoing study by one of the authors, researching an ACT protocol for OCD, many participants found this simple exercise to be one of the most useful in the protocol. This makes sense, as one way of viewing OCD is as an inability to notice the difference between five-senses experience and mental or inner experience, resulting in compulsive attempts to respond to provocative mental or inner experiences as if they were five-senses experiences to be banished. For example, the thought of contamination can lead to behavior appropriate to a five-senses experience of contamination. Further, when clients perform their compulsions, they're so caught up in their mental experience that subsequently they are unable to discriminate whether they experienced performing the compulsion with their five senses or simply thought they performed the compulsion, which in turns feeds obsessional doubt. This way of approaching OCD can be quite liberating for clinicians, because it can free them from having to go into the content of obsessive thoughts while still allowing them to effectively help their clients free themselves from taking their thoughts literally.

Hooks

As mentioned in the introduction, cognitive defusion is one of the six processes targeted by ACT. It was initially referred to as deliteralization. This made-up word proved unwieldy, so the ACT community soon settled on another made-up word: defusion. Defusion is the process of noticing thoughts, emotions, and other types of inner experience, rather than being so caught up in them that they seem to be welded to us, as if we were seeing the world through the lens of our thoughts and emotions. In other words, defusion is about gaining perspective on our inner experience and noticing the difference between five-senses and mental experience.

An initial step in defusion is to gain a bit of distance from the content of our inner experience so we can notice that experience for what it is—passing thoughts and emotions—rather than for what it says it is. In cognitive therapy, this is known as distancing. Yet ACT doesn't stop at distancing. As a functional contextual approach, ACT always looks for the function of events in context. So defusion isn't confined to just noticing and distancing from inner content; it also involves noticing the behaviors that arise as a result of being fused. Then we can notice if the behavior that arises when we're fused with our inner content is consistent with our values and workable.

Presenting the Hooks Metaphor

In our clinical practice, we've found that the Hooks metaphor is ideal for matrix defusion work. This metaphor illuminates how one single process can make us forget the difference between the world of five-senses experience and the world of inner experience and also casts light on the behaviors that can lead to. The following dialogue illustrates how you can introduce this metaphor.

Therapist: I don't know if you know anything about fishing. I don't, so if you do, jump in and correct me if I talk nonsense.

Client: My dad used to fish.

Therapist: Great. I understand it's not the hook that makes the fish bite, it's the bait that's wrapped around the hook, but I'll call it a hook for short. I understand that different species of fish bite different hooks.

Client: Right.

Therapist: And I've heard that the same fish will bite different hooks in different contexts. For example, you'd use a different hook if fishing for salmon in the ocean than you would when the same kind of salmon is swimming up a river.

Client: Yes.

Therapist: I've also heard that the same fish in the same lake will bite different hooks depending on the season.

Client: Really?

Therapist: So they say. But how do fish notice that they've bitten a hook?

Client: It hurts?

Therapist: Well, they could bite other things that would also hurt, yet they wouldn't be hooked. They could even bite a hook that wasn't attached to a fishing line and also wouldn't get hooked. So how do they notice they're hooked?

Client: Because they get pulled...

Therapist: Right. Because they get pulled in a different direction than they were swimming before the hook showed up and they bit. We're similar to fish in this way. Under the surface of the horizontal line of the matrix, all sorts of hooks can show up. Our hooks can be made up of any number of things: thoughts, emotions, bodily sensations, memories, stories, images, or sometimes even five-senses experience: something we see or hear. We can even get hooked by thoughts about who or what is important. Sometimes we get hooked by a combination of things. And like fish, we can better notice that we're hooked by looking at what we do next— which direction we swim in—than by looking at the hook itself.

Client:	Okay…
Therapist:	As we're talking about hooks, can you start noticing some of your hooks and what you do next when you're hooked?
Client:	I think so.
Therapist:	Great. Don't tell me what you came up with just yet. Let's consider fish again for a minute. If fish could notice that hooks are hooks, what would we see them do?
Client:	Not bite… Swim around, I guess.
Therapist:	Most likely they'd just swim around and continue swimming toward whatever they were swimming toward before the hook showed up. Now tell me, would they ever need to get rid of hooks?
Client:	No.
Therapist:	Understand hooks?
Client:	No.
Therapist:	Analyze hooks?
Client:	No.
Therapist:	Explain hooks?
Client:	No.
Therapist:	Identify who's holding the fishing line?
Client:	No.
Therapist:	Or know for how many generations their species has been biting this particular hook?
Client:	No.
Therapist:	So it would be enough for them to just notice hooks as hooks?
Client:	I guess.
Therapist:	Well here's the good news: we can learn to recognize hooks as hooks. And this we do by simply noticing hooks and what we do next. After all, fishing is not catching. So although all sorts of experiences can hook us, including five-senses experience, we can learn to recognize hooks and choose not to bite.

Using the Hooks Worksheet

We've developed the Hooks Worksheet to help clients notice what tends to hook them and how getting hooked influences their behavior. (The worksheet is available for download at http://www.newharbinger.com/33605.) After introducing the Hooks metaphor, show clients the hooks worksheet and invite them to fill it in before your next session. Alternatively, you can fill it in with them during the current session. The worksheet depicts ten fishing lines complete with hooks and bait. Ask clients to write on the bait what hooks them and on the line what they do next.

HOOKS WORKSHEET Write your hooks on the bait, and on the fishing line, write what you do next. For example you might write "Anger" on a worm, then write "Raise my voice and leave" on the line.

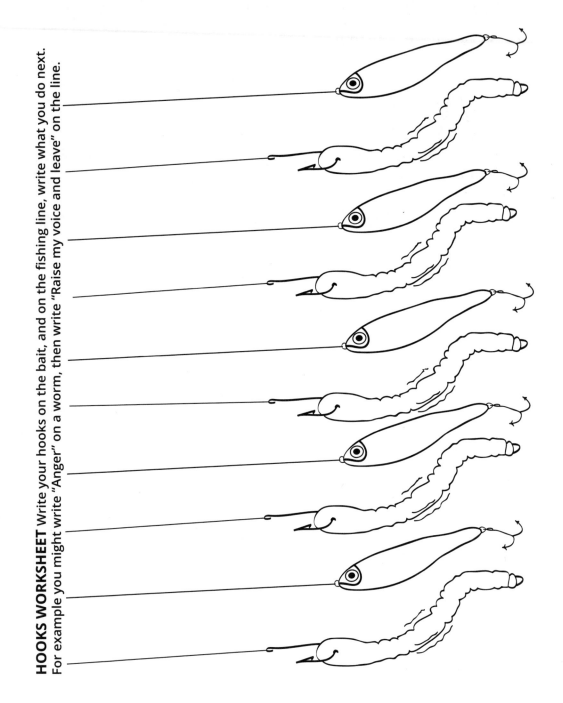

The Essential Guide to the ACT Matrix

In most cases, clients will write some sort of inner experience on the bait and an observable behavior on the line. So, for example, "Irritation" would go on the bait and "Shouting at my children" on the line. However, what clients write will reflect either their experience or their current sorting abilities. For example, a client may write the thought "I'll never succeed" on the bait, and on the line write "I ruminate," which may not be outwardly observable.

Occasionally, clients may write their observable behavior (for example, "criticizing") on the bait and their inner experience (perhaps "irritation") on the line. Rather than seeing this as a problem in which clients are sorting incorrectly, view it as an opportunity to help them refine their sorting skills by practicing noticing the difference between inner experience and outwardly observable behavior.

Sometimes clients may experience that what hooks them is not an inner experience but something they perceive through their five senses (as alluded to in the preceding dialogue). Of course, sometimes things in the world of five-senses experience can be extremely powerful hooks. With some clients, you may want to mention how the mere sight of a yummy cookie, a glass of wine, or a wrap of drugs may function as a hook. In other cases, clients may specify an outer experience. For example, a woman might put "My husband criticizing me" on the bait, rather than an aspect of her inner experience that gets her hooked, such as anger or feeling that she isn't good enough.

Use the worksheet flexibly. It isn't necessary for clients to identify or describe the inner experience that constitutes the genuine hook. There is no "genuine" hook, just getting hooked or not. So in the preceding example, the client need not describe her inner experience of her spouse making critical comments; she can still notice that she gets hooked and behaves differently than she would if she hadn't gotten hooked.

Sometimes clients may get hooked by the thought that you're suggesting their hooks are all in the head and not real. Instead of getting hooked by such reactions, invite these clients to write their "real" hooks on the bait on the worksheet. You could then say something like "Some hooks appear in our five-senses experience. Besides, to me, no experience is more or less real than any other. Thoughts, emotions, and five-senses experience are just different types of real experience."

Catch-and-Release Fishing

Recently, we've refined the Hooks metaphor to incorporate the experience of our colleague Hank Robb, an accomplished ACT therapist and a keen angler. These days, we always wrap up presentation of the Hooks metaphor by saying something along the following lines.

Therapist: A lot of what I know about fishing I've learned from a friend who's been fishing since he was a kid. Nowadays, he mostly releases the fish he catches. Over time, he's noticed two behavior changes. His own behavior has changed, as he's started using barbless hooks. This makes it easier to unhook fish and throw them back in the water. But the most noticeable behavior change has been in the fish in some of the streams where he fishes. In the past, the moment fish got hooked, they would fight and flail to the point of being nearly dead from exhaustion when they were finally reeled to shore. These days, some fish don't fight or pull against the hook as much. They seem to just wait to be released. This makes for very boring fishing because the fish don't fight. The only explanation my friend can think of is the fish have become so accustomed to getting hooked and then being released that they've learned that the fastest way to get back to swimming toward whatever they want is to not fight against the hook.

This presentation has proven most useful with clients who get hooked by noticing that they get hooked. In this way, noticing the thought *I got hooked again* can function as a hook for clients who are easily hooked by self-blame. It also suggests a way out of getting hooked: not fighting the hook or the observation that they will inevitably get hooked. In such cases, you might say (provided this is true of you) something along the following lines.

Therapist: When I first heard this, I realized that this was a story about the kind of fish I am. I notice that I still bite pretty much the same hooks I've always bitten. The difference is that I now more quickly notice that I got hooked, and when I do, I simply fight less against the hook. And I've noticed that the less I flail, the faster I get back to swimming toward whatever I was swimming toward.

You can then simply invite clients to notice their hooks and what they do next, including noticing when they flail against the hook after they get hooked and when they don't and whether that makes a difference.

The Hooky Words Game

We recommend concluding the discussion of hooks with a game that can help clients get unhooked. It involves looking at words in terms of how "hooky" they are and how they can get us hooked. Here's an example of how you might present it.

Therapist: Words can easily hook us and then pull us toward doing things we wouldn't otherwise have done. And when we're hooked, some words are so hooky that they really pull at us. It's as if once they've hooked us, they pull and get into us like the purple unicorn. In fact, the more we try to move away from them, the deeper they hook us. You can notice how hooky words can be by noticing how it feels to just hear them or read them. Is it okay if I throw some words around so we can look at how hooky they feel to us?

To begin the game, invite the client to rate how hooky each word you'll offer is on a scale of 0 to 5, where 0 is not at all hooky and 5 is extremely hooky. Then throw out several words, some that are likely to hook the client and others that are more neutral, pausing after each to allow the client to rate it. Then invite the client to throw some of her own hooky words into the ring. Some hooky words that have come up a lot when playing this game are: loser, suicide, cutting, anorexia, addict, unlovable, hopeless, depression, fear, anxiety, stupid, therapy, drugs, alcohol, mother, father, trauma, sex, rejection, borderline, difficult, oppositional, narcissistic, and acronyms like ADHD and OCD.

The hooky words game can be an effective way to get clients and therapists alike to interact more flexibly with words that can hook them. It's also a playful and highly participative way to promote defusion, as the simple act of noticing one's response creates some distance. Sorting the words into categories of hooky and nonhooky and then assigning ratings to them then furthers the process of defusion.

Step 3 Home Practice: Noticing Hooks and What You Do Next

As always in matrix work, the home practice is to practice noticing. Invite clients to continue noticing their toward and away moves, perhaps ramping up the frequency to more than once a day for clients who are readily engaging in the practice. Of course, many clients will do this on their own; however, some may benefit from a gentle nudge. Also ask clients to notice hooks, whether they bite, and if so, what they do next and whether they notice a difference between when they flail against the hook versus when they don't. You can give clients the Hooks Worksheet to record their experience with this over the coming days. If it seems helpful for a given client, you might supplement this home practice with the exercise for sorting five-senses and mental experience for one minute a day, as described earlier in this chapter.

How to Notice and Flexibly Sidestep Potential Traps

This session is generally well received by clients. The experiential exploration of the effectiveness of trying to control inner experience can be very helpful in setting up a workable discrimination of which aspects of experience can be controlled and which may become more problematic if we attempt to control them. Even so, there are a few potential traps and sticky points, including getting hooked by hooks!

Clients Saying They Can Control Thoughts

Some clients may hold a firm belief that thoughts, emotions, and other inner experiences can be controlled. The trap here would be trying to argue with the client's assertions or appearing skeptical of them. One reason to steer clear of this trap is that research indicates it is indeed possible to repress thoughts—at least for a while (Wenzlaff & Wegner, 2000). In such cases, aim for a stance of open curiosity. Ask these clients whether controlling inner experience feels effortful and whether it works when they really want it to work. Remember, matrix work is all about pointing to clients' experience. Gently acknowledging what the client noticed—whatever that may be—generally serves to set up a context of further noticing. Within that context, it's common for clients to revisit this topic in the future and share that they noticed that it's not so easy to suppress thoughts or emotions.

Qualifying the context can also be helpful. You can note that, in your experience, it's possible to control or suppress thoughts and emotions when they're not too sticky, but when the going gets tough, people usually notice that controlling their inner experience is a lot more difficult. You might also revisit the shark pool exercise and how it demonstrates that if you're hooked by the idea that the slightest sign of fear means death, then a high level of fear becomes highly probable. If, on the other hand, it's just a matter of seeing things slightly differently on a good day, controlling inner experience may indeed prove easier. But once again, be sure to orient clients to their own experience, rather than trying to fit their experience into a theory or model. You can then simply invite them to notice the contexts in which suppressing or changing thoughts and emotions works with little effort and the contexts in which it's harder.

Getting Hooked by Hooks

One of the potential pitfalls of using the Hooks metaphor is that clients can look at hooks in a mechanistic fashion. In such cases, clients may demand a precise definition of hooks, demanding to know exactly what they are, when you're actually inviting them to recognize hooks more through the behaviors they engage in next (a functional definition). Repeating something like "A hook can be whatever makes you bite" can only go so far. Here again, an attitude of openness and curiosity can help you sidestep this trap. Give these clients a simple example of a hook, like fear or wanting to be right, and then ask whether they've ever noticed being pulled to do something they wouldn't have done were it not for fear or a desire to be right. It can be helpful to share one of your own experiences of getting hooked.

Limiting Hooks to Unwanted Inner Experience

Hooks are whatever makes us bite. In presenting hooks, it's generally best to start with pointing to unwanted inner experience—the stuff in the bottom left quadrant. However, be sure to mention that hooks can show up just about anywhere: in the lower right quadrant or even in five-senses experience. Sometimes they can even show up in the form of wanting to move toward some particular inner experience, such as relaxation, feeling good, or being right. The key to becoming adept at identifying hooks isn't in localizing where in the matrix they show up, but whether they cause us to behave differently than we would have if we hadn't gotten hooked.

Focusing on Hooks Rather Than Getting Hooked

The fact that hooks show up isn't a problem. In fact, it's a given. The point of the work is to help clients notice when hooks show up and then choose what they wish to do next. Therefore, it isn't necessarily problematic that behavior follows the appearance of a hook. What matters is whether the person is able to choose behavior to move toward who or what is important, even in the presence of hooks. For example, losing a loved one can be a powerful hook. The behavior that follows could take many forms: crying, not crying, withdrawing, connecting more closely with others, or drinking to excess, to name a few. If the client values crying and showing emotion to acknowledge the loss, that wouldn't be hooked behavior, even if it feels painful or is an expression of negative emotion.

It's best to steer clear of questions such as "Would you have done that in the absence of the hook?" Instead, inquire about instances where clients seem to have gotten hooked—perhaps drinking to excess when sadness about the loss of a loved one shows up. Try the formulation "Would you have done that if you hadn't gotten hooked?" This may work better to focus clients' attention on what they do when actually hooked.

Getting Hooked by Other People Getting Hooked

Hooks commonly show up as we witness other people's behavior. Imagine you're driving to work on a beautiful sunny morning when a teenage driver cuts you off and nearly crashes into you. You might get hooked by what just happened, and everything else will disappear. Fear may hook you, as may thoughts about how dangerous and careless teenage drivers are. When you eventually get to work, you may still be hooked by what happened and perhaps launch into an angry tirade about how teenage brains are unfit for driving. You got hooked by someone else's behavior. Chances are, if that teenage driver could notice her hooks, she might notice that her dangerous driving occurred after she'd gotten hooked.

Clients often report getting hooked by other people's behavior. That's perfectly natural. So in the above example, you could simply write "almost being sideswiped by a teenage driver" on the bait in the Hooks Worksheet.

Frequently Asked Questions

What if clients claim they can control their inner experience?

As discussed, in these cases it's generally best to validate that some people do indeed report that they are able to control thoughts and emotions. Then, as recommended, inquire about how easy it is for the client to do that and whether she's noticed any side effects or costs, being sure to do so with an attitude of genuine curiosity. Most clients will report that doing so is quite draining. You can then suggest that there may be a more efficient way to deal with unwanted thoughts and feelings and move on to looking at emotions through the metaphor of a lie detector. If clients report that controlling thoughts or emotions isn't difficult or effortful, gently ask whether they've tried to apply these strategies to their presenting problem. You can even invite them to try some of those control strategies and report how it went in the next session.

Won't clients feel invalidated by discussion of hooks?

When presenting hooks, it's crucial to do so from a profoundly validating standpoint. Hooks don't just make people bite; they can be intensely painful. Intensely distressing experiences such as trauma memories, feeling abandoned or unloved, panic sensations, or pain can hook clients and therapists alike.

Therefore, as pointed out in the section on sidestepping potential traps, it's important to separate hooks from getting hooked. For example, in the presence of sadness, a client may want to cry, as this is how the person she wants to be would respond to sadness. In this context, crying isn't an instance of getting hooked. For this person, getting hooked by sadness might instead mean hiding her sadness and pretending everything is fine.

When working with hooks, be sure to mention how intensely painful some hooks can be. Then provide a couple of examples of painful hooks, along with examples of behavior that illustrate getting hooked versus not getting hooked. For example, in the presence of a painful memory about being assaulted, getting hooked could lead a person to attempt to suppress that memory and avoid going out, whereas not biting might mean taking some time to validate how painful the memory is and then going out as planned.

Going Deeper

To dive deeper and uncover some of the processes at work in step 3, we'll take a closer look at the paradoxical effects of cognitive control efforts. We'll also consider cognitive fusion in some detail and look at how working with hooks can foster helpful transformations of functions.

The Paradoxical Effects of Cognitive Control Efforts

In the late 1980s, groundbreaking work by Daniel Wegner and his team at Harvard documented the paradoxical effects of thought suppression (Wegner, Schneider, Carter, & White, 1987). Instructions to suppress a thought result in multiplication of the suppressed thought. These effects carry over into emotion suppression (Cioffi & Holloway, 1993). In fact, thoughts suppressed in the presence of a particular emotion are more likely to reappear when the same emotion shows up, even in a different context

(Wenzlaff & Wegner, 2000). To be fair, within this body of research some people report that they are able to suppress thoughts successfully.

However, the moment they stop trying to suppress a thought, it bounces back. Occasionally, you may have clients who report that they are able to not think of a purple unicorn. You can validate that, perhaps saying something like "It's great that you noticed that you could not think of the unicorn. Some people can do that. Did it take a lot of energy? Many people find it's like holding a ball underwater. And the bigger the ball, the more effort it takes. What happens when you stop holding it down? It bounces up and can even splash you." Steer clear of invalidating clients' claims or appearing to disbelieve them. After all, each person is the expert in noticing her own inner experience. The more you recognize and reinforce this expertise, the more likely it is that your clients will become flexible and nondefensive in their noticing.

In addition to studying thought suppression, Wegner's team looked at behavior suppression in an intriguing study in which they asked participants to hold a pendulum steady over the center of a grid etched into a horizontal glass plate (Wegner, Ansfield, & Pilloff, 1998). A video camera underneath the plate recorded the pendulum movements. In one condition they asked participants not to move the pendulum. The recorded paths deviated pretty much randomly from the crosshair. In the next condition, participants were asked not to move the pendulum along one of the axes of the grid. The fluctuations were largely in the direction participants had been instructed not to move the pendulum. The researchers then ran the same two conditions while also adding cognitive load by asking participants to mentally count backward from 3,000 by steps of 3. The deviations increased, especially in the suppressed direction. This last study points to the importance of learning to do new behaviors to replace problematic behaviors, rather than simply trying to not do the problematic behaviors. In matrix work, we never invite clients to not engage in away moves; instead, we invite them to notice what toward moves they could engage in.

With those studies in mind, consider this: What proportion of your clients ask you to help them with not thinking X, not feeling Y, not doing Z, or some combination of these three goals? We've asked this question of over three thousand participants in our training workshops, and based on their replies, the proportion falls somewhere between 99 and 100 percent. You could say that, as clinicians, we don't have the easiest job in the world!

So, dear reader, over the past week how many times have you noticed your mind telling you not to think, feel, or do something?

Defusion

One of the main targets of ACT is fusion, characterized by excessive dominance of behavior by narrow verbal functions over other available functions. In other words, fusion happens when we get hooked by what our minds are saying. Once we start using language, most of us largely spend our time in our head. The running commentary of the mind rarely stops. It comments on everything, including virtually every moment of our five-senses experience.

That said, our verbal abilities are one of our greatest assets as a species, and they've given us incomparable control over the world outside the skin. So they aren't the enemy—but they aren't always our friend. They can trip us up time and again as we get hooked by rigid verbal rules and act without regard for what the situation affords or the wider impact of our behavior. A lot of away moves come down to fusion in the sense that they arise due to the application of rigid rules, such as "I must not feel this" or "If I think this, I must do that."

ACT places a great deal of emphasis on freeing people from excessive dominance of these verbal functions, and ACT texts contain many defusion exercises and metaphors that can help put some distance between individuals and their thoughts. As people learn to create that space (which is an act of perspective taking), they greatly increase their ability to choose their behavior.

We've found it helpful to think of defusion work as occurring in two main stages. The first is identifying inner content and distancing oneself from it: recognizing thoughts as simply thoughts, emotions as simply emotions, and bodily sensations as simply bodily sensations, rather than imperious commands to behave in a certain way. The second stage is identifying the function of the content in the context of interest: what we do next when this stuff shows up and whether it's what we would have chosen to do. If it isn't, we know we've been hooked.

The way step 3 works with hooks can accomplish a lot of the ACT defusion work, given that it comprises these two steps. Asking what hooks show up helps clients identify what sort of content they tend to fuse with. Then, asking what they do next elucidates the function of the hook in the context of interest. This is why it's crucial to eventually ask whether the behavior that follows the hook showing up is what clients would have done had they not gotten hooked. This allows clients to sort behavior between that which is under the inflexible control of hooks (fused content) and a broader, more flexible behavioral repertoire.

Initially, it's usually best to stay with the yes/no question "Is this what you would have done had you not gotten hooked?" rather than immediately moving to more open questions such as "What else could you have done?" or "What would the person you want to be have done?" (a topic we'll address in chapter 4). The yes/no formulation helps clients learn to reliably notice that they got hooked, as indicated by the fact that they suddenly found themselves being pulled in a different direction than they were swimming before the hook showed up. Until they can notice this, they're likely to get hooked without noticing that it's happened, so their answers to the latter questions are likely to be a function of getting hooked.

Consider the example of a client getting hooked by anger in interactions with her teenage children. Her kids regularly behave in ways that her mind tells her are disrespectful, and it makes her angry to experience that. When anger shows up, she gets hooked and starts yelling at them. When asked whether yelling is what she would have done, she can readily answer no, especially because she's noticed that yelling doesn't work to get her kids to behave more respectfully. However, if she were also initially asked what else she could have done, she might answer that respect is essential in families, that kids need to have respect to succeed in life, that disrespect should be met with consequences, and so on. She could still be so hooked that she'd flail against the hook rather than consider what other behaviors are available if she isn't hooked by anger. This is why we typically cover those latter questions, aimed at values-consistent behavior, in step 4, when clients are formally introduced to verbal aikido.

In the Frame

Exploring the effectiveness of control efforts in the inner world versus the outer world sets up a frame of opposition between the two. This can help reduce the avoidance functions associated with aversive inner experience. As inner experience becomes framed with stuff that gets stickier the more one attempts to control it, derived aversive functions can attach to control attempts, reducing their short-term attractiveness.

Inviting clients to notice hooks and what they do next brings in deictic framing— the ability to take perspective on one's own experience. The ability to notice hooks in turn opens up the possibility of broader tracking. For example, prior to being framed in this way, a hook might have hitherto functioned as a rule: "I do this (away) behavior because I have this thought or emotion, or because that's the kind of person I am." Clients might also engage in narrow avoidant tracking, such as noticing that away moves serve to reduce their immediate discomfort. Noticing hooks can help set the stage for tracking more broadly, including tracking congruence with their desired behavior and then with their values. Such tracking can help clients discriminate between behavior under the control of inflexible rules and values-based action stemming from broader appetitive functions. All of this can arise from simply asking clients to notice whether what they do after they notice getting hooked is what they would have done had they not gotten hooked.

Step 3 Checklist

Use this checklist (available for download at http://www.newharbinger.com /33605) to guide your practice of the strategies outlined in this chapter.

What I did

☐ I debriefed the home practice in a flexible way.

☐ I set up a context in which my client could compare humanity's progress in controlling five-senses experience versus inner experience.

☐ I invited my client to experientially explore the effectiveness of thought suppression.

☐ I invited my client to notice how often her mind tells her to not think of something and to think of something else instead.

☐ I invited my client to experientially explore the effectiveness of emotion suppression.

☐ I invited my client to notice how often her mind tells her to not feel something and to feel something else instead.

☐ I invited my client to practice sorting five-senses and mental experience.

☐ I presented the Hooks metaphor, noting how different fish bite different hooks and how the same fish will bite different hooks in different contexts or seasons.

☐ I asked my client whether, if fish could notice hooks as hooks, they would need to get rid of hooks, fight hooks, explain hooks, understand hooks, and so on.

☐ I presented the idea of catch-and-release fishing and invited my client to notice whether she fights against hooks after biting them.

☐ I invited my client to fill in the Hooks Worksheet.

☐ As a home practice exercise, I invited my client to notice hooks, whether she bites, and if so, what she does next.

☐ I shared some of my hooks in a way that didn't put me at center stage.

What I didn't overdo

☐ Presenting these exercises and metaphor as a didactic monologue, rather than inviting client participation through dialogue

☐ Presenting not biting hooks as easy to do

CHAPTER 4

Step 4: Verbal Aikido

From a matrix point of view, we typically get stuck because we aren't paying attention to all the relevant aspects of our context in a given situation. Moreover, we tend to get stuck because we bite hooks and then behave differently than we would have had we not gotten hooked. When we notice hooks, we gain some precious distance from them and can choose our behavior, whereas previously our only option seemed to be blindly biting hooks. Then we can turn toward other important aspects of the context, particularly what those other choices might be. What would the person we want to be do? And who or what is important about being able to do that? Deliberately paying attention to these aspects of our experience is crucial for getting unhooked and choosing values-congruent actions.

Keeping all of these elements of the context in mind may seem like an effortful endeavor that we must practice deliberately. However, the goal is not to get people to identify all the potential hooks moment to moment and then calculate what a toward move would be in each situation. Rather, the goal is to help people notice how it feels to move toward values, much as we learn to notice how it feels to find, keep, and regain our balance on a bicycle. We don't do that by calculating our center of gravity moment-to-moment or by determining how much kinetic force to apply in what direction to regain our balance. If that were necessary, only a handful of people could ever ride a bicycle, and none of them would have fun cycling.

So another important step in matrix work is to help people learn how it feels to engage in toward moves and how this differs from the feel of engaging in away moves. And as with learning to ride a bike, this can be an experience akin to noticing when they find their balance, noticing when they lose it, and noticing what it takes to regain it. Furthermore, just as being balanced on a bike is more appealing than losing balance, moving toward who or what is important is more appetitive than moving away from what we don't want to think and feel. This is what step 4 is about. We call it verbal aikido, and it's a highly effective skill for getting unstuck.

Because verbal aikido is so central to matrix work, we'll begin with a general overview of this approach before describing how to use it with clients.

The Basics of Verbal Aikido

Aikido stands out from most martial arts in its purpose. It's not about defeating one's opponent; it's about rolling with the energy of the attack to bring about peace and harmony. Aikido practice emphasizes being present in the moment, avoiding struggle, and taking resistance as a gift.

The term "verbal aikido" and some of the particulars of this practice were incorporated into matrix work after a number of aikido practitioners noted that aspects of matrix work reminded them of the physical practice of aikido. They were referring to how matrix practitioners deftly step out of the way of provocative words that clients throw into the ring—or, to stick with martial arts imagery, the words clients throw onto the mat. After stepping out of the way by not getting hooked by the content of the words, matrix practitioners simply ask clients to sort their words into the matrix.

The essence of aikido practice is being open to new learning. The first goal of the trainer is to get the student involved in the practice, which is accomplished by making the student feel that anything done in practice is useful for learning. Similarly, in matrix work we try to communicate that anything clients say, think, or feel is welcome and can be useful in the context of therapy. Using "Yes, and..." responses is at the heart of verbal aikido, as it redirects the mind's energy into noticing and sorting, thereby helping clients unhook from unworkable stories and behaviors.

Yessing

In contrast with boxing or karate, aikido doesn't involve launching, blocking, or avoiding attacks; rather, it's a practice of aligning with the other person's energy and redirecting it. To do that, the practitioner must be centered, notice the struggle and not get sucked into it, and take what is offered as an invitation to practice moving toward the other person. Similarly, the "Yes, and..." practice involves accepting and building on what clients offer. In this practice, you accept (by saying "yes") whatever behavior clients offer before inviting them (by adding "and") to do some sorting on the matrix. You seek to remain fully present in the moment, noticing any struggle and validating any resistance, both clients' and your own, and utilizing whatever clients offer as an opportunity for them to practice sorting. This trains clients in the psychological flexibility point of view, from which there are no right or wrong answers, just behaviors that are more or less workable.

Contrast this to more traditional cognitive behavioral therapy. In CBT, therapy can be about challenging and changing clients' thoughts and beliefs, which can easily turn into verbal wrestling or boxing (although highly skilled Socratic questioning can come close to the fluid stance of verbal aikido). In traditional CBT, "Yes, but..." is more common than "Yes, and...." And "Yes butting" can quickly turn into a head-butting game of opposites where client and therapist find themselves at loggerheads.

Yessing, when genuine, is at the heart of acceptance, whereas butting is at the heart of resistance and conflict. In the original ACT book, *Acceptance and Commitment*

Therapy (1999), Hayes, Strosahl, and Wilson recommended encouraging clients to practice replacing "but" with "and," particularly in the context of thoughts and stories that were keeping them stuck ("I want to give more presentations, but I'm too anxious"). For matrix work, we believe that taking a profoundly yessing stance with clients greatly diminishes their resistance to adopting the psychological flexibility point of view. When practicing verbal aikido, don't seek to move clients from one place to another; just invite them to notice and sort. The simple phrase "yes, and" does just that. Saying "yes" is an effective way of providing validation and promoting acceptance, and "and" offers an effective invitation to open to something new, fostering flexibility.

Sorting in the Present Moment

Being centered in aikido is similar to being present in therapy. Instead of thinking about how you might block your opponent's next attack and preparing your next move, you can choose to be present, making room for the experience that arises from the other person's invitation. Similarly, working with the matrix invites you to be present and make room for clients' inner experiences, which can then be sorted.

As mentioned previously, sometimes your mind will tell you that clients are sorting wrong. At such times, you might get hooked into trying to explain the matrix to help them sort "correctly." If you do this, you'll step away from aikido and slip toward wrestling. One of the most common hooks for both therapists and clients is the idea that therapists are there to solve problems. When we bite this hook, clients can readily turn into problems to solve—and nobody wants to be a problem to be solved (Sandoz, Wilson, & DuFrene, 2011).

Noticing what hooks you as a therapist and how those hooks can pull you away from a flexible aikido stance is a crucial skill. Sorting isn't for judging, analyzing, evaluating, or solving problems. Rather, the aim is to help therapists and clients alike notice present-moment experience in a less verbal way. It can also help therapists remain in a stance of being a witness of the human being in front of us.

Validation

In aikido, you pay constant attention to the other person's movements and body, not just because this allows you to neutralize incoming attacks, but so you can take care of the other person when you align and redirect the energy of the attack. To do this, you practice looking at the situation from the attacker's point of view.

Likewise, in therapy the clinician displays an understanding of the client's point of view, thus creating a safe context in which learning can take place. This is especially true when practicing basic verbal aikido moves. Among the many descriptions of how to create a context that takes the client's perspective into account and promotes learning, we've found the description of validation steps and levels in dialectical behavior therapy offered by Kelly Koerner (2012) particularly helpful. In this section, we'll present our interpretation of these, geared for use with the matrix.

Validation can be thought of as comprising two components: displaying empathy for what the client is experiencing, and verbally expressing that the client's perspective is valid and understandable. Validating is key to building a strong alliance, and it can also be an effective intervention. Through validation, you create space for clients' deep emotions, making it easier for them to contact and stay with uncomfortable experiences, thereby reducing their drive to move away from such experiences.

It should come as no surprise that practicing verbal aikido with the matrix depends on the therapist taking a validating stance. As we've emphasized repeatedly, this work is most effective when therapists invite clients to sort from their own point of view. Here are three effective ways to enhance your verbal aikido through validation.

Recognize the client's point of view as it is. This is best done by reflecting the client's experience. Kelly Koerner (2012) offers this effective metaphor: A man calls you asking for directions, and you tell him to turn right toward the freeway ramp. At the other end of the line, he insists that the sign to the freeway ramp is pointing left. Until you've met and reflected his experience, perhaps with words such as "Okay, so from where you're standing the freeway ramp sign is pointing left," there's no chance he'll listen to you. It wouldn't make sense for him to. When interventions don't get off the ground—including matrix interventions—it's often because therapists insist that clients should take their advice before meeting clients where they are.

Recognize the importance of the client's felt experience without buying into the content of that experience. When clients are sharing content that reduces their flexibility, validate that you get what they feel or think without buying into the content of what they're saying. For example, if a client says, "My life is hell because my wife has stopped loving me," buying into that content might lead to a response like "It's really painful that your wife doesn't love you anymore." Such an answer can validate what your client is saying, but it also supports the client's inflexible framing of the problem as "my wife has stopped loving me." A more flexible response might take the form "It's really painful to feel that your wife doesn't love you anymore." This targets the feelings without hooking into content. At worst your client might answer, "It's not what I feel. It's a fact!" Again, you can respond flexibly, this time by saying, "It's really painful to live through that." This validates the experience without reinforcing an inflexible description of the situation.

Validate a lot early in treatment, then validate less. This technique reflects a gradual shaping of clients' self-validation abilities. Create a warm and supportive interpersonal context to support training psychological flexibility. Gradually, as clients learn to self-validate through the course of therapy, you can shift to a more natural conversational style. Whenever things get sticky, try going back to validation before you try anything else.

Marsha Linehan (1997) outlined six levels of validation and recommended that, whenever feasible, therapists should aim to validate at the highest level possible. In keeping with the spirit of the aikido metaphor, we've outlined these as belt colors.

White belt: The basic skill at this level is to listen with mindful attention. Be fully present to the client and the exchange. Though this may seem obvious, there will be times when you'll find it hard to be present, especially when clients launch into a well-worn stuck story. In such cases, it may be a good idea to gently ask for permission to interrupt. Then invite clients to notice their matrix, notice hooks, practice the verbal aikido moves (which you'll learn shortly), or simply take a breather so the two of you can reconnect.

Yellow belt: The skill at this level is reflecting clients' experience in their own words, from their point of view. Some therapists reformulate what clients say in elaborate ways. Though this may sometimes be effective, it's more likely to make clients interact with your words, rather than contemplating their own experience and noticing that you got what they were saying. We've found that using the client's own words whenever possible is often highly effective—even going so far as to repeat their words in the first person. For example, if a client says, "I'm such a loser; I don't know if I can ever get better," you could reflect, "So, 'I'm such a loser; I don't know if I can ever get better' shows up." When you do change clients' wordings, keep an eye out for whether they start responding to your reformulations, rather than to their own experience.

Orange belt: At this level, you seek to reflect unformulated feelings, which may be obscured to clients. Let's say a client named Juan is recounting a work meeting during which his boss told him his performance had been poor lately, and Juan felt insulted by the way his boss said this in front of the whole team. He says he felt really angry, but listening to him, you notice some sadness. You could then say, "Yes, and did any sadness show up too?" Alternatively, imagine that, recounting the same event, Juan says he felt sad when his boss put him down in front of the whole team. If you detect glimmerings of anger, you could then seek to reflect these unexpressed feelings: "Yes, and did any anger show up too?" Another approach is to help clients formulate their implicit feelings and then reflect them. Let your own feelings be the guide in the interpretations you put forth. The key here is to hold whatever you share lightly. Remember, there is no right or wrong, and you can never know clients' experience better than they can. What makes your interpretations useful isn't their "objective truth"; they are only useful insofar as they can help clients better notice their own experience. Plus, when you demonstrate letting go of your thoughts if they don't resonate with your client's experience, you provide an effective model for not biting hooks.

Green belt: At this level, you reflect how clients' behavior makes sense in terms of their personal history. Although you can do effective matrix work without knowing much about a client's personal history, in most cases stuck patterns arose early, initially serving as perfectly adaptive responses to aversive situations. Then, over time, these patterns may have gotten the client stuck. Reflecting to clients how their behavior makes sense in terms of what they've experienced can provide strong validation. Returning to our example, imagine that you know Juan had a difficult relationship with his dad growing up and that he regularly felt mocked and criticized at the dinner table. Unable to talk back to his dad, he developed the habit of retreating to his room. When he tells you that after his boss criticized him he took refuge in the bathroom, you can reflect how, in light of his family history, it makes sense that he would have done that.

Blue belt: At this level, you reflect how clients' behavior made sense in context. ACT practitioners might find this challenging, hesitating to validate away moves. After all, ACT is about helping clients engage in toward moves, so it's reasonable to worry that validating away moves could inadvertently reinforce them. However, away moves are rarely inherently stupid. They generally make sense in the context in which they take place. As discussed in chapter 2, many of these behaviors work in the short term, allowing people to move away from unwanted inner experience. However, away moves are also generally a sign that clients weren't able to notice and choose other actions. In any case, it can be highly validating for clients to hear that you get how an away move made sense, as that may have been all they could think of doing at that time, and because it was probably effective in bringing some short-term relief. In short, biting hooks makes sense. So in Juan's case, you could say something like "I get it. You got hooked by feeling insulted and left the room. At the time, that's all you could see to do. Plus, I imagine you may have initially felt some relief after leaving the room."

Brown belt: At this level, you validate clients as they are: fully human, flaws and all. From an ACT perspective, we are all in the same boat, sailing in the same ocean of words. We all get hooked and stuck at times, and nobody is broken or defective. The more therapists openly sort with their own matrix and help clients sort with theirs, the more our common humanity shines through. ACT therapists work from a position of radical equality with clients and establish the therapy context as a place of learning for both client and therapist. One of the most effective ways to convey this is through disclosing your own matrix to clients. Returning to our example, let's say that you share Juan's tendency to get hooked by feeling insulted. At this level of validation, you can share that and let Juan know that when you feel slighted, you sometimes do things like leave the room. This form of self-disclosure, when done in the client's service and not to put your own experience at center stage, provides a very high level of validation. More generally, unconditional positive regard and a heartfelt warm manner will go a long way toward creating an optimal context for client learning.

Black belt: After practicing the skills outlined at all the preceding levels, you can integrate them in a flexible way that constantly adapts to the changing context of therapy. Be present, mindfully reflect clients' experience in their own words, reflect unstated feelings whenever you feel this could be helpful, and show that you get how their away moves make sense in the context of their life history and in the contexts in which they engage in them. Finally, remember that we're all in the same boat, and share your own matrix as needed. Each client, each session, and each time you speak can offer a new opportunity for you to engage in a toward move—moving toward the therapist you want to be.

The levels of validation we've outlined spell out, in a detailed way, what we mean by "yessing." They will be most useful to you if you approach them as flexible guidelines rather than rigid rules. We chose to outline them in some detail because, in our work as trainers and supervisors, we noticed that clinicians can easily get stuck when using the matrix if they neglect to do so from a stance of deep validation. Without validation and yessing, the learning context can quickly become aversive to clients, in which case verbal aikido moves may fall flat or even become aversive. By deliberately bringing a validating stance to your work, especially early on in therapy, you will create an optimal context in which clients can experiment with and practice psychological flexibility skills.

Steering Clear of Verbal Wrestling

As mentioned, physical aikido stands apart from other, related disciplines by deliberately steering clear of struggling. As you engage in the moves we'll set forth in this chapter, be alert for times when your approach may engender struggling and result in verbal wrestling. To help you notice the distinction, we'll provide a series of potential dialogues with our hypothetical client Juan. See if you can identify which exchanges are closer to verbal aikido and which are closer to verbal wrestling.

Exchange A

Therapist: What did you notice when your boss said that?

Client: I started thinking what a jerk he was and what a loser I am.

Therapist: Yes, and what does being a loser mean to you?

Client: I don't know. Someone who can't cut it and will never be able to make it. Someone who everybody makes fun of and nobody respects.

Therapist: That's tough. And have you ever had any success at work that your boss has praised?

Exchange B

Therapist: What did you notice when your boss said that?

Client: I started thinking what a jerk he was and what a loser I am.

Therapist: Yes, and what do you usually do when this stuff shows up?

Client: I isolate myself. I shut down and leave.

Therapist: That sounds hard. And what would the person you want to be do?

Exchange C

Client: If I look back, I can't think of a single time my boss has recognized my work.

Therapist: Oh wow, that must be painful. But are you sure? You've been there for over ten years. There must have been a few times when things were going well.

Client: I guess so. But right now I can't remember any.

Therapist: I understand. It's often like this when we're upset. We tend to generalize.

Client: It's hard not to generalize when it happens every time.

Therapist: I understand that this is all very upsetting to you.

Exchange D

Client: If I look back, I can't think of a single time my boss has recognized my work.

Therapist: That sounds really painful. It really sucks to feel that way.

Client: Sure does!

Therapist: It sounds like feeling unrecognized might be a big hook for you.

Client: Uh-huh.

Therapist: Yes, and what do you do when this hook shows up? Do you notice that you bite?

Client: You bet!

Therapist: And what do you do next?

Client: I usually withdraw.

Therapist: That makes perfect sense—as if the hook is so large that it's kind of hard to see anything else. Plus, withdrawing can give you instant relief.

Client: Yeah, but what can I do?

Therapist: It's not easy. I can also get hooked by the feeling that I can never get it right, and then I tend to withdraw too.

Client: You do?

Therapist: Yes, sometimes. And what would the person you want to be do when this hook shows up?

Although the therapist attempts to be validating in exchanges A and C, you can probably notice those two exchanges quickly slipping toward verbal wrestling. This happens because the therapist tries to interact with the content of what the client is saying, rather than sidestepping the content and going with the client's felt experience. In this context, validation is likely to fall flat. In exchanges B and D, the therapist practices verbal aikido consistently and validates at different levels, which supports Juan in turning with curiosity toward what else he could have done.

Home Practice Debrief

Now we'll turn to conducting step 4 and presenting verbal aikido to clients. As in previous sessions, you can start with the short settling-in exercise from chapter 2. Alternatively, you can go straight to debriefing the step 3 home practice: noticing toward and away moves, as well as hooks that showed up and what clients did next. For clients who filled out the Hooks Worksheet, you can go over what they've written. If you invited the client to practice sorting five-senses experience versus inner experience, debrief that as well. Throughout, reinforce clients for noticing and encourage them to continue practicing.

Introducing Verbal Aikido

One of the noticeable effects of sticky thoughts, feelings, and emotions—those that get us hooked—is to pull us away from the broader context and trap us up in our heads, where we're more likely to seek to apply general and generally rigid, unworkable rules. Verbal aikido can help us get back in touch with the relevant aspects of the context and help us move toward workability. Therefore, verbal aikido is truly the heart of matrix work.

As a matrix practitioner, you'll practice verbal aikido from the moment you begin an intervention till the moment your work is done. Although some practitioners apply aikido without explaining what they are doing, we've found it extremely effective to tell clients about verbal aikido and explicitly teach them the basic moves.

You can introduce verbal aikido by saying that a number of people who are familiar with both aikido and the matrix have noticed strong similarities between the two. For clients who don't know much about aikido, which may be most of them, you can say something along the following lines.

Therapist: Aikido differs from other martial arts in that its purpose is not to defeat one's opponent, but to create peace and harmony by engaging in moves that deflect the energy of the attack. With the matrix, we practice verbal aikido, meaning we go with the energy of whatever our minds or emotions throw at us, doing so in a way that brings our minds and ourselves to a state of peace and harmony, which it does by helping us become more effective in moving toward who or what is important to us.

The Verbal Aikido Worksheet

To help clients learn and practice verbal aikido, we've developed the Verbal Aikido Worksheet (available for download at http://www.newharbinger.com/33605). Based on the matrix diagram, it includes various questions pointing to different quadrants of the matrix.

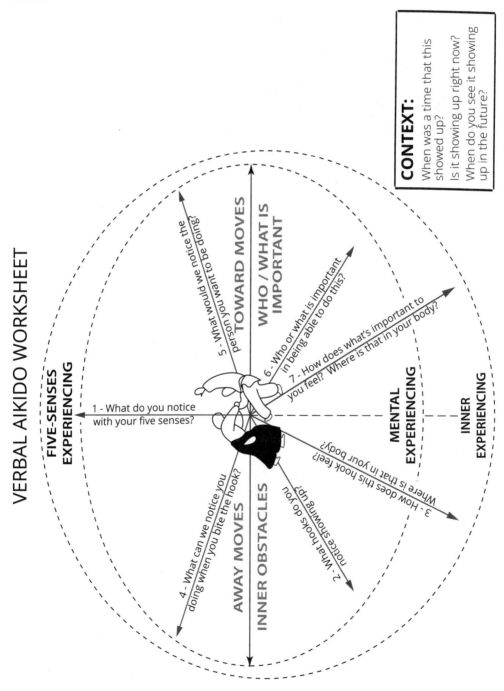

Pointing to Different Aspects of Inner Experience

As you can see, on the Verbal Aikido Worksheet, we've introduced something new: layers, or circles, the inner one labeled "mental experiencing" and the outer one labeled "inner experiencing." As you can see, in the lower half of the matrix, two of the verbal aikido questions point only to "mental experiencing": What hooks show up? And who or what is important? The other two questions in the lower half extend fully into "inner experiencing." This allows practitioners to direct questions at how it *feels* to get hooked and stuck in away moves and how it *feels* to contact who or what is important and engage in toward moves. It also allows clients to respond in ways that are less tied to verbal experience.

In addition, these questions help clients tune in to a highly important aspect of their context that often goes unnoticed: their bodily state and how it feels to experience whatever they're experiencing in the moment. Many people have lost contact with that aspect of their context or have never learned to notice and name it. The two questions that extend into "inner experiencing" are therefore useful for helping people notice and connect with the bodily aspects of their context.

All of that said, this division into layers doesn't imply that we think there's a fundamental difference in nature between mental and inner experience. However, by orienting clients' attention to their experience of how toward and away moves feel and where those physical sensations show up, they gradually come to notice the difference between toward and away in a less verbal way. Ultimately, this helps them tune in to how it feels to shift toward living more on the right side of the matrix. Again, it's akin to paying attention to how it feels to ride a bike. Words are a poor vehicle for capturing how it feels to notice when you're in balance, when you're beginning to lose your balance, and what you do to regain it. This is why as we move further into matrix work, we increasingly want to draw clients' attention to less wordy aspects of their experience, which we designate here as "inner experience." That said, we are fully aware that a large part of that inner experience is shaped by verbal functions.

Introducing the Worksheet

After you've introduced the general idea of verbal aikido, you can offer clients the worksheet, explaining that there are seven basic verbal aikido moves and that the worksheet maps them onto a matrix in the form of questions. Then ask clients if they'd be willing to practice the basic verbal aikido moves with you.

In our experience, clients unfailingly agree to try those moves at least once. Once they agree, invite them to choose something important, difficult, or both difficult and important that they'd like to talk about. Mention that, like all martial arts, aikido is initially best practiced in a specific area—one designated for that purpose. For verbal aikido, that means choosing a concrete situation. The three questions in the box in the lower right corner of the worksheet can help with this:

When was a time that this showed up?

Is it showing up right now?

When do you see this showing up in the future?

Practicing the Moves

You're now ready to practice the basic verbal aikido moves by exploring the questions on the worksheet, initially proceeding through them in numerical order. As you can see, many of these questions inquire about aspects of the matrix already touched upon in steps 1 through 3, so we won't explain them individually. Rather, we'll offer an example of using this approach with a client.

In the following dialogue, the clinician is guiding Lisa through her first verbal aikido practice. Lisa is a thirty-five-year-old mother of two young children whose life has been severely limited by a crippling fear of panic attacks. In response to this fear, she's come to avoid most activities unless an adult family member is present or in the immediate neighborhood. In her quest to get rid of panic symptoms, she's previously tried a number of courses of CBT and, more recently, a more traditional ACT therapy. In this dialogue, and on the example worksheet provided in this chapter, we've used numbers to refer to the questions in order to facilitate presenting the dialogue. In actual practice, the numbers aren't used, as the eventual aim is for clients to learn to engage in these moves flexibly, in a way that fits their current situation. Therefore, the downloadable worksheet also lacks the numbers used here.

Therapist: What would you like us to talk about?

Client: About my fear of panic symptoms, of course.

Therapist: Great. So when was a time that it showed up?

Client: Driving my daughter to day care on my own two days ago.

Therapist: *(Points to question 1.)* Where were you at the moment you want us to look at? See, I'm asking you a five-senses question.

Client: In my car at the stoplight.

Therapist: Can you see what was around you?

Client: There's a park on one side and shops on the other.

Therapist: Great! *(Points to question 2.)* And what hooks did you notice showing up?

Client: Is that where you start?

Therapist: Yes, I started with five-senses questions, and now we're moving to hooks.

Client:	Is there an order to it?
Therapist:	For this first practice, we can do it this way, and then you'll find your own way of using those moves. So did you notice a hook showing up?
Client:	Yes, the thought "I'm afraid I'll panic."
Therapist:	Ouch! That sounds like a painful hook. *(Points to question 3.)* How did that feel in your body? Where was that?
Client:	In my head, dizziness, then *(pointing to her chest)* chest pressure.
Therapist:	Okay, so pressure in your chest, dizziness in your head. And did you bite the hook?
Client:	Yes, I did bite.
Therapist:	*(Points to question 4.)* And what did you do?
Client:	I called my husband.
Therapist:	Okay, good. *(Points to question 5.)* And what would the person you want to be have done? What would we have seen her do?
Client:	Nothing. She would have kept driving to day care.
Therapist:	*(Points to question 6.)* And what is important to you in being able to continue driving in a situation like this?
Client:	Being independent and being able to do things for my daughter.
Therapist:	Okay, good. *(Points to question 7.)* How does it feel when you say it's important to you to be independent and to do things for your daughter?
Client:	It's very important!
Therapist:	Yes, and how does it feel? Where is that in your body?
Client:	It feels, hmm… I feel depressed!
Therapist:	Oh wow. Where is that in your body? Where is it most intense?
Client:	In my heart, I guess.
Therapist:	Can you point to the place?
Client:	*(Points to her upper left chest.)* Here.
Therapist:	Okay, good.

When Lisa looked at that last question (How does what's important to you feel?), it looked to the therapist as though she was getting hooked. In these kinds of situations, you may wish to invite clients to engage in a second round of verbal aikido practice. It's quite common for clients to get hooked when they look at who or what is important to them in being able to behave like the person they want to be in a situation in which they commonly get hooked and can't engage in a toward move. Remember, hooks can at times also show up on the right-hand side (and then quickly move to the left). In such cases, it can be useful to invite clients to a second round of verbal aikido. Note, however, that verbal aikido practice should be aimed at getting clients to practice, not at making them feel a particular way—for example, feeling good when they contact who or what is important to them. In Lisa's case, the therapist chose to work around the hook that appeared to show up, resulting in the exchange that follows.

Therapist: So now we've completed our first practice of the basic verbal aikido moves. Was that okay? I can see it was painful at times. Would you be willing to go for a second round?

Client: Okay.

Therapist: Great. *(Points to question 2.)* You said, "I feel depressed." Could that be a hook for you?

Client: Hmm… Yes.

Therapist: Good. *(Points to question 3.)* How does it feel when "I feel depressed" shows up?

Client: Like I'm gonna go down a dark road. *(Giggles.)*

Therapist: That sounds hard. *(Points to question 3 again.)* And how does it feel in your body when you notice the thought "I'm gonna go down a dark road" showing up?

Client: Sadness.

Therapist: *(Points to question 3 again.)* Yes, and show me where that is in your body. If you're not sure, just point randomly.

Client: *(Points toward her eyes and forehead.)* In my eyes, and in my head.

Therapist: Okay, good. *(Points to question 4.)* And what do we see you do when you bite that hook?

Client: Distraction. Well, I was going to say, "Think about something else," but you couldn't see me do that. So I'll say, "Do something else."

Therapist: Okay, and do you have an example of what we could see you do on a video monitor?

Client:	Call a friend.
Therapist:	Excellent! *(Points to question 5.)* And what would the person you want to be do in a situation like this, when depression shows up along with the thought "I'm gonna go down a dark road"?
Client:	Just continue doing what I was doing.
Therapist:	For example?
Client:	Pick up my daughter.
Therapist:	Okay, cool. What's important to you in being able to pick up your daughter?
Client:	Being there for her.
Therapist:	Being there for her. Okay. And how does it feel when you say it's important to you to be there for her?
Client:	It makes me feel good.
Therapist:	Okay. Where is that in your body?
Client:	Where is that in my body? In my head, I guess.
Therapist:	Okay. Show me where in your head.
Client:	Hmm… No, not in my head. *(Points to her chest and giggles.)* In my heart.
Therapist:	Cool! So you've just practiced a couple of rounds of the basic verbal aikido moves. How was that for you?
Client:	It was good, because it's only just noticing.
Therapist:	Great. Excellent.
Client:	I mean, it's different from having to answer questions like "Oh, and why are you feeling depressed?" It's just noticing. *(Pauses and heaves a sigh.)* Yeah.
Therapist:	Great. Now I'm going to say something that's probably going to shock your mind. I hope you don't run away just because I say it. Are you willing to hear me say it?
Client:	*(Giggles.)* Hmm… I don't know. Okay, yeah.
Therapist:	You know, what we do here is basically just learning to ask ourselves these seven questions in any stuck situation. Many people find that they're able to learn these seven questions fairly quickly. And I'm going to

be here to help you notice them in the situations where you get stuck. So between now and next week, see if you can notice opportunities to explore these seven questions.

In her second pass at the basic verbal aikido moves, Lisa noticed some warm feelings in her heart when she contacted how important it is for her to be there for her daughter. That's fine and may even be an indication that she's now better able to contact her deeper values, even in a stuck context. However, practicing verbal aikido is about flexible noticing, not about getting anywhere, much less about getting to "good" feelings or the "right" way to sort one's experience, or stating rigid rules about how the person one wants to be would have acted. At heart, it is an exercise in noticing all the relevant aspects of the context in situations where we get hooked, stuck, or both. It's important to remember that and to be sure clients understand it; otherwise you or your clients may ask and respond to these questions under the control of rigid verbal rules.

Practicing on the Hooks That Show Up in the Practice

As clients practice verbal aikido around a given context, they're likely to hit spots of inflexibility, which often show up as hooks. In our experience, these hooks may well show up on the right-hand side of the matrix, as happened to Lisa. Whether these hooks appear on the right-hand side or left-hand side, it can be extremely helpful to clients to zoom in on those points of inflexibility for some focused verbal aikido practice.

Because the questions about hooks are in the lower left quadrant, it may initially seem counterintuitive that hooks can show up on the right-hand side, so let's take a closer look at that. Clients who aren't yet adept at noticing hooks and what they do next can easily get stuck when pondering the question "What would the person you want to be have done?" Occasionally, clients may say that there was nothing else they could have done, given what they were thinking and feeling in the situation. This is a sign that they haven't been able to distance from their hooks enough to identify whether certain thoughts and emotions can lead them to behave differently than they would have if they didn't get hooked. In such cases, validate their experience and gently invite them to imagine that nothing had shown up in the bottom left quadrant. Although hooks can show up pretty much anywhere—bottom right, bottom left, or in five-senses experience—those that are easiest for clients to relate to generally show up in the bottom left, as unwanted inner experience. So when clients have trouble identifying what the person they want to be would have done, it's often helpful to have them imagine what they would have done if unwanted inner experience hadn't shown up. This can allow them to see what else they might have done.

Another place where hooks can commonly show up is when pondering the question "Who or what is important in being able to do this?" At first clients may give left-hand answers, such as "It's important to not feel anxiety." In most cases, there's no need to do anything with such answers, as any large hook can be addressed through the next move: "How does that importance feel, and where does it show up in your body?" It's not uncommon for clients to answer this question with stories rather than by naming feelings. In fact, this is the primary reason why we ask them to point to where the feelings show up physically. This orients them to more direct experience, rather than mental processing.

How Many Times to Practice Verbal Aikido

Typically, going through a round of verbal aikido questions takes just a few minutes. And with many clients, you'll start to see more psychological flexibility right away. If not, continue to practice the basic moves a few times. At the end of each round, pause to debrief the experience, then ask clients whether they'd like to practice another round. Two or three rounds usually suffice. With time, you'll develop a feel for how many initial rounds are optimal for each particular client.

One way to invite clients to further practice is to ask them what they'd like to practice on next, whether other aspects of the same situation or a different situation altogether. In some cases, as with Lisa, you may feel that it would be helpful to do some extra practice on what showed up in the first round. If so, just ask for permission before proceeding.

Practicing on Different Time Points of the Same Situation

It can be quite effective to practice the basic verbal aikido moves on different time points of a given situation. Consider Jenny, a thirteen-year-old junior high student struggling with assertiveness at school and in shared custody arrangements with her dad, who's remarrying. When we introduced verbal aikido, she chose to practice around a recent instance of working on a team class project and in which she got hooked by anger, a familiar hook for her that regularly shows up both at home and at school. When she bites that hook, she tends to shut down and not attempt to express her needs.

In the first round of verbal aikido, painful hooks showed up in the lower right quadrant when we asked, "How does that importance feel, and where does it show up in your body?" So we asked her if she was willing to do a second round of verbal aikido around the painful feelings of sadness that had shown up when she'd looked at the bottom right-hand side in the first round. Then, when we focused on those hooks, she was able to connect with how important it is for her to learn and have fun. She found that second round harder. Then she said, "Wait—there's more," and moved on to the next time she got stuck while working on the same project with her class team.

Soon Jenny was able to notice the anger hook showing up regularly. She could also point to the place in her belly where she felt it and notice that what she does when she gets hooked is say nothing. Moving to the questions on the right side, she saw that the

Jenny she wants to be would speak up and take an active role in situations that matter to her. This is what was important to her in the situations she chose for verbal aikido practice. Interestingly, when we had presented the matrix to her in the first session, Jenny had identified "Not saying anything" as one of her main away moves. Ultimately, although verbal aikido brought up some challenging content for Jenny, she enjoyed practicing the basic moves and eagerly took the printed worksheet home to guide her in further practice. She also noticed that she found it easier to express her needs both at school and at home.

Step 4 Home Practice: Engaging in Verbal Aikido

For step 4 home practice, invite clients to practice verbal aikido in a variety of situations. To maximize their success, emphasize that it will take practice to get to the point where they can successfully engage in verbal aikido in real time. You might recommend that they begin by practicing verbal aikido retrospectively, looking at a stuck situation from the past. Next, they might practice prospectively, contemplating future situations where they might get stuck. These consciously chosen practices will help them access their verbal aikido moves in real-time stuck situations. Of course, if you feel a particular client would benefit from continuing with any of the previous home practice exercises, recommend those as well. And as ever, invite clients to continue noticing toward and away moves as often as they possibly can.

Before concluding the session, cast your future work together as an ongoing verbal aikido practice. Explain that future sessions will focus on helping them hone their verbal aikido moves in the different stuck situations they may encounter.

How to Notice and Flexibly Sidestep Potential Traps

Verbal aikido may seem simple, but it isn't easy. You must engage in regular and deliberate practice in order to become an adept and flexible practitioner. And as you start out, you're likely to encounter various traps that are all too easy to fall into. Here are a few of the most common, along with advice on how to flexibly sidestep them.

Being Too Abstract

A common pitfall among therapists who are just beginning to use verbal aikido is not making sure clients focus on concrete situations. If you start with a general problem, say battling obsessions, rather than a concrete situation that can be identified in space and time, such as compulsively checking the stove last night, you run a high risk of getting lost in abstractions. In the land of generalities the mind reigns supreme, and bringing flexibility to this realm, which is so dominated by rigid abstractions, requires highly honed verbal aikido skills.

Asking clients to choose a particular situation to practice on, as described earlier in this chapter, will go a long way toward circumventing this trap. Even so, clients may respond in more general terms. When this happens, ask as many five-senses questions as it takes for clients to connect to a specific, concrete situation. When they do, you'll notice that your shared verbal aikido practice becomes immeasurably more flexible.

In the second or third round of practice with a given client, you might notice that it becomes easier to practice on more general or abstract situations. However, should you subsequently feel that the practice gets stuck, it may be because the discussion has become too abstract. In this case, once again ask the client to supply a concrete example, using five-senses questions as needed.

Not Focusing on Observable Behavior

When asked about what they do when they get hooked, or about what the person they want to be would do, clients may provide answers other than descriptions of observable behavior. For example, a client might say that when he bites the hook he ruminates, or that the person he wants to be wouldn't feel anxious. In such cases, as with presenting the matrix, simply ask clients what they could be seen doing on a video monitor or what you could have seen them doing had you been there.

Trying to Get to a Predetermined Outcome

When clients practice verbal aikido, they may develop flexibility quickly. However, this isn't always the case. For some clients, a number of rounds of basic moves may be necessary before they reach a more flexible stance. In such cases, it's especially important to remember that practicing verbal aikido is more about the practice itself than about reaching a particular outcome.

In these situations, your mind may offer evaluations, perhaps that the client is making mistakes, or that you are. Mistakes aren't a problem; they're an inevitable and precious part of learning. If clients get stuck or stumble, see if you can receive that as part of the practice, perhaps by offering a spoken acknowledgment of how difficult these moves can be at first and then gently inviting them to continue. If you feel that you yourself have stumbled, this could provide a wonderful opportunity to practice verbal aikido on your own situation. Here's an example.

Therapist: So when you get hooked, you start drinking. And what would the person you want to be do?

Client: I don't know. Drink, I guess. I know you think that's really bad and I'm just making my situation worse, but that's all I know to do. Besides, I love the taste of a good wine.

Therapist:	Yes, but it gets you stuck.
Client:	Well, I'll never get better then.
Therapist:	Wait. I noticed that I just stopped practicing the basic moves there. Can we slow down and look at what just happened for me?
Client:	Sure.
Therapist:	Okay. (*Points to the Verbal Aikido Worksheet.*) So I got hooked by the idea that I'm here to prevent you from drinking when you know that drinking is bad for you. I felt anxious and impatient, and I noticed some constriction in my chest here (*pointing to her chest*). And when I got hooked, you saw me try to force you to see that drinking is necessarily biting the hook for you. And off to the races I go…
Client:	That's okay. I also get hooked.

Using Verbal Aikido to Get to Feeling Good

Another potential trap is using verbal aikido as a way to help clients feel good. In verbal aikido practice, it's not uncommon for clients to experience warm feelings when they notice how it feels to contact what's important to them in being able to behave like the person they want to be. As pleasant as this is, it's more of a side effect, not the primary goal of verbal aikido. As in ACT more generally, verbal aikido isn't about feeling better; it's about better feeling what there is to feel in a given situation—and about noticing the difference between how away moves and toward moves feel. Also remember that it may sometimes feel good to engage in away moves or feel bad to engage in toward moves. One of the most important goals of verbal aikido is to notice the difference between these two discriminations: feeling good and feeling bad, versus the feel of moving toward and the feel of moving away.

Frequently Asked Questions

Aren't the verbal aikido questions too limiting?

Some practitioners initially rebel at the idea that therapy might basically come down to seven questions asked in relation to two lines drawn on a piece of paper. Benjamin Schoendorff, who came up with these questions, initially got hooked by similar thoughts and started giving trainees the worksheet with the printed questions while recommending that they subtly modify the wording so their clients wouldn't notice that they were repeatedly using the same basic moves. Then a trainee at a workshop said he was going to print the questions and simply ask clients if they'd willing to talk about whatever they chose using just those questions. A few months later Benjamin himself tried it in a couples session. It worked so well that he never looked back. The questions help point therapists' and clients' attention to all the relevant aspects of the context, thereby increasing flexibility.

Aren't these questions too superficial?

At first we got hooked by this question too. Then we saw that many clients contact deep emotions while practicing these basic moves, at times tearing up. This allowed us to notice that the questions allow clients to go as deep as they choose to go, thereby giving them more control over the process. That helps them feel safe and take considered risks, which makes the questions highly workable.

A client once remarked that because she knew what questions would come up, she felt free to go deeper than she would have had her therapists' questions felt like prying into her private world. Because these questions allow clients to titrate how deeply they look as they practice the basic moves, they not only stay in control of the situation but also learn to choose ways to contact their deeper feelings and values that are workable for them.

Do I really have to show these questions to my clients?

Some clinicians have a hard time showing these questions to their clients. Their minds tell them that their clients may rebel, end the session, or refuse to do the exercise. You may wonder whether it would be better to just use the questions without openly showing them to clients. You may, of course, do that. We've worked both ways—showing the questions and not showing them—and our experience is that showing them tends to greatly speed the process and give clients more control over it.

What if clients don't know how their hooks feel, how what's important feels, or where those feelings show up in their body?

We've found that an effective way to deal with such situations is to simply ask clients to point randomly to any part of their body. The very worst that's happened as a result was that a client pointed to her left knee as the place where anger showed up. With time, she became increasingly skilled at noticing where feelings of getting hooked or moving toward something important showed up in her body, and having pointed at her knee became a running joke between her and her therapist.

What if these questions don't solve a client's problems?

Using the basic verbal aikido moves isn't about solving problems; it's about helping people acquire flexibility in the situations where they get stuck. The "solution" that we train is psychological flexibility—the ability to choose to do what's important in the presence of inner obstacles. When clients are stuck, the problem is rarely that they don't know what else they could do; rather, it's typically that they don't know what else they could do in the presence of these obstacles. Flexing by paying attention to all aspects of their experience (that is, noticing the entirety of their matrix) in the situations where they get stuck will help them arrive at their own solutions. And solutions that people arrive at on their own are more likely to endure in the long term than ready-made solutions others suggest to them. From the matrix point of view, the role of the therapist is to create a context that fosters psychological flexibility, not to give clients solutions.

What if clients don't get unstuck using these questions?

You may have gotten stuck on our answer to the previous question, so here's a follow-up. The fact is, sometimes clients don't initially get unstuck by simply using these questions. This isn't necessarily a problem. The basic verbal aikido moves will eventually help anyone flex in situations where they get stuck. For some clients who are very stuck or who find themselves in very sticky situations, deliberate practice will be required for flexibility to show up. Gradually, it will. From the moment you introduce these questions, you'll be able to refer back to them anytime. And because it's easy to practice them in a few minutes, you should be able to invite clients to engage in a few rounds each session. In fact, once you've introduced the basic verbal aikido moves to a client, we recommend that you keep on using these questions in all future sessions, whenever workable.

What if I feel stupid using these questions?

At first you may well feel stupid. We did. However, once we noticed the powerful effect these questions had on our clients, and the even more powerful effect of simply showing them the questions and inviting them to practice verbal aikido, we figured feeling stupid every now and again was a price we were willing to pay to help our clients get unstuck faster.

Won't clients think I'm a robot, just parroting these questions?

The best way to find out is to ask them. We've found that working from a context of choice is central. Asking clients for permission to use these questions goes a long way toward making the questions interesting and even appetitive. Of course, no technique replaces paying close attention to the effects of your behavior on your clients or, said another way, the functions of your interactions. If you notice that asking these questions evokes a strong aversive reaction in a given client, be sure to ask him what's going on and what you could do to better meet his needs.

If you notice that asking these questions is evoking a strong reaction in many of your clients, consider whether you can improve the validating quality of the context within which you ask them. You may want to review the section on validation earlier in this chapter. Then deliberately practice validation at every level possible, bringing particular attention to meeting clients in their experience, validating their felt experience without buying into their content, validating how their behavior makes sense in the context, and validating them as human beings, including sharing some of your own experience to validate that we are all in the same boat, sailing the verbal ocean.

Going Deeper

In this section, we discuss some of the behavioral principles at work in verbal aikido and the relational frames that may be activated by this practice. We'll also explore why we've come to see verbal aikido as perhaps the ultimate aim of ACT treatment.

Increasing Flexible Tracking

We believe that practicing verbal aikido helps people unhook from pliantly following rules or counterpliantly disobeying them. It also helps them broaden their tracking abilities beyond narrowly noticing that away moves can temporarily reduce discomfort. Because the questions promote contacting and noticing the broader aspects of the context in any given situation, they effectively promote flexible tracking: noticing much of what is present, particularly the broad consequences of any given behavior.

Augmenting

The verbal aikido moves help clients consider who or what is important in being able to engage in a chosen behavior—whether they actually engage in the behavior or simply identify it as what the person they want to be would do. In either case, this renders the behavior more salient and increases the probability that clients will engage in it. Contacting who or what is important within the behavior is an effective way of contacting values, which tend to serve as *augmentals*: verbally constructed reinforcers that increase the probability of engaging in toward moves, persisting in them, and gradually refining them. We make use of augmentals to train psychological flexibility, and in our experience, one of the most powerful augmentals is asking oneself the simple question "What would the person I want to be do?" Of course, nothing is 100 percent effective for 100 percent of people 100 percent of the time. However, when you ask this question with genuine curiosity (rather than from an ulterior motive of getting clients to do something other than their stuck behavior), it can make behavior that was low in probability become more salient and more appetitive. In other words, the question "What would the person you want to be do?" is one of the most effective augmentals you can use in clinical practice. (We'll discuss augmenting in greater depth in chapter 5.)

In the Frame

The verbal aikido questions can be powerful cues to increase derived relational responding under the appetitive control of values. As with all matrix practice, using these questions cues perspective taking and deictic framing. Even when practiced in real time, these questions help clients gain a me-there-then perspective on their experience, as noticed from the perspective of I-here-now. In other words, the questions evoke framing events with respect to the basic deictic relations that lie at the heart of perspective-taking: I-here-now contrasted with you-there-then.

Noticing hooks as hooks can transform and weaken their controlling function on away moves. Meanwhile, when clients notice what the person they want to be would do, who or what is important in being able to do that, and how that importance feels, this can strengthen the appetitive functions of toward moves, making them more probable.

Other forms of relational framing may also be cued. For example, framing toward and away moves in opposition may produce conditions that increase the derivation of aversive functions to away moves and cue the derivation of appetitive functions to toward moves. Depending on a client's learning history and the features of the situation you're working with, many different forms of derived relational responding might take place. The visual cue of the matrix can help ensure that they are held within a broad network of relations that tends to enhance appetitive functions and render toward moves more probable.

Verbal Aikido as the Ultimate Aim of ACT Treatment

The more we've worked with verbal aikido, the more we've come to think that perhaps the ultimate aim of ACT interventions, whether in clinical or other settings, is to help people engage in some equivalent to the basic verbal aikido moves in any stuck situation. If this initially sounds a bit strange, consider the many ways in which verbal aikido captures the fundamentals of ACT. The basic moves help clients make contact with the present moment by orienting them to all significant aspects of context: five-senses experience, inner experience (which includes their learning history), and the function of their behaviors in the context of interest. On the left-hand side, verbal aikido also explores experiential avoidance (leading to away moves) and cognitive fusion (leading to hooked behavior). And on the right-hand side, it explores committed action (toward moves) and values (who or what is important).

Finally, noticing and answering the questions—in other words, engaging in verbal aikido—is, in essence, an act of perspective taking. This not only creates distance from content that may hook clients and promotes acceptance, but also helps them take the perspective of I-here-now viewing the experience of me-there-then. From that perspective, they can take a more empathetic stance toward their experience and difficulties. They can also notice that choices are available to them even in highly stuck situations. In sum, practicing verbal aikido can be an effective way of looking at things from a functional contextual point of view, seeing the big picture, and increasing workability.

Of course, all of this doesn't lead to instant dissolution of all present and future difficulties and an eternal state of infinite bliss. Far from it. It simply offers an effective way to get unstuck and tone up psychological flexibility. That flexibility may not stop people from getting stuck again. After all, getting stuck is almost inevitable due to the stickiness of words and the attraction of away moves. However, the flexibility engendered by verbal aikido will increase the likelihood of getting unstuck faster.

Ending Treatment: Getting Unstuck Faster

Once clients become flexible in their practice of verbal aikido, they will have acquired most of the skills they need to get unstuck faster in important situations. Whereas initially they may well have felt as though they had no choice but to behave in unworkable ways, they can now notice more options and choices. Soon they'll notice themselves choosing toward moves over away moves in formerly stuck situations.

A fairly large proportion of our clients (somewhat less than 40 percent as a rough clinical estimate) learn enough in the first four steps to get unstuck in most situations. For these clients, we might end treatment in a final session after completing step 4, rather than going on to the material outlined in chapters 5 and 6. To wrap up, we begin the final session by asking clients what they noticed in their home practice of the verbal aikido. We then invite them to practice the moves in session, using a couple of concrete situations. If they can use the questions to increase flexibility pretty much unaided, we then rephrase the psychological flexibility question posed when wrapping up the presentation of the point of view in step 1: "Do you feel that you are now better able to choose to do what's important to you even in the presence of inner obstacles?" If they answer yes, we suggest that our work together might be coming to an end and offer to meet again in a month or two to check in on how things are going.

At this point, it can be a good idea to mention that therapy isn't about never getting stuck again, sharing that even on a good day, we ourselves notice getting stuck at least once. You might proffer that therapy is more about learning to notice when we get stuck and then getting unstuck faster, and that getting unstuck is a skill that requires lifelong practice, ideally in real-life settings. This may also be a good time to share some appreciation with clients, mentioning what they've accomplished, the progress they've made, times when they touched you, and what you wish for them going forward.

Of course, some of your clients won't develop sufficient psychological flexibility using just the first four steps. As you might have guessed, in our clinical experience, this is the case for a good 60 percent of clients. For these clients, continue with steps 5 and 6, which target self-compassion and perspective-taking skills, as outlined in the next two chapters.

Step 4 Checklist

Use this checklist (available for download at http://www.newharbinger.com /33605) to guide your practice of the strategies outlined in this chapter.

What I did

- ☐ I debriefed the home practice in a flexible way.
- ☐ I practiced the first level of validation by being fully present to my client.
- ☐ I practiced reflecting what my client said in terms close to those he used.
- ☐ I expressed how my client's away moves made sense in terms of his personal history.
- ☐ I expressed how my client's away moves made sense in the context in which he found himself.
- ☐ I showed the client my own matrix or personal experience to illustrate how we are all in the same boat.
- ☐ I presented verbal aikido in a general way before inviting my client to a round of the basic moves.
- ☐ I shared the Verbal Aikido Worksheet with my client.
- ☐ I invited my client to choose a past situation to work with using the basic verbal aikido moves.
- ☐ I made sure we worked with a concrete, specific context, asking five-senses questions as needed.
- ☐ After a first round of the basic moves, I asked my client how it was for him and offered to practice additional rounds as needed.
- ☐ I invited my client to share how hooks and importance felt and asked him to point to where in his body he noticed these feelings.
- ☐ When posing the questions in the upper half of the matrix, I asked my client to describe observable behaviors.
- ☐ As a home practice exercise, I invited my client to engage in the basic verbal aikido moves.

What I didn't overdo

- ☐ Asking the verbal aikido questions without validating my client's feelings and how difficult things might have been for him
- ☐ Getting hooked by content and veering away from the verbal aikido questions

CHAPTER 5

Step 5: Training Self-Compassion

Some clients have trouble practicing the basic verbal aikido moves. This often comes from not being able to notice hooks before biting them and subsequently getting caught in stuck loops that make it difficult for them to notice the right-hand side of their matrix.

Faced with a threat, all animals, humans included, tend to respond in one of three ways: by fighting, fleeing, or freezing. Some people tend to bite certain hooks so quickly that they activate the fight, flight, or freeze response before they can notice anything in a useful way. In these cases, their relationship with a given hook is so antagonistic or avoidant that their capacity to notice the hook as a hook is impaired, so hooked behavior almost inevitably follows the appearance of the hook itself. This happens when wounds are deep, and also when people get hooked by self-blame, self-judgment, or a pervasively narrowing self-story. More concisely and technically, the function of the hook is to narrow the range of responses to a reduced, inflexible, and unworkable repertoire.

In such cases, we've found that training self-compassion can help change the behavior that follows the appearance of the hook. In this chapter, we offer an effective self-compassion exercise (previously presented in Tirch, Schoendorff, & Silberstein, 2014), along with a few modifications that can help both clients and clinicians drop their inner struggle and choose the road of inner reconciliation.

Opening the Session

As in previous sessions, you may wish to start with a short settling-in exercise, followed by debriefing any and all noticing by simply reinforcing whatever clients noticed. Next, as in previous sessions, debrief clients' home practice. Ask them what toward and away moves they noticed. Also ask whether they practiced the verbal aikido moves. As mentioned at the end of the previous chapter, not all clients will experience increased flexibility after just a week or so of practicing verbal aikido. In fact a majority won't. Be prepared for that. You'll know whether clients need more training if they find it difficult to answer the basic verbal aikido questions in a flexible way. Of course, those who didn't practice verbal aikido since the previous session are also likely to need more training. Some clients will say something like "It was just too hard" before recounting how they got stuck again. It's important to validate such clients and assure them that they aren't alone in finding it difficult to practice verbal aikido. Then share that in this session the two of you will work on an exercise that will make practicing verbal aikido easier (the Mother Cat Exercise, which is the primary focus of this step). In fact, even for clients who have experienced increased flexibility, you may still choose to offer the exercise in this step.

The Mother Cat Exercise

Words and learning histories can easily stand in the way of adopting a gentler perspective on one's own experience. To weaken their power we use the Mother Cat Exercise, a metaphor-based approach aimed at connecting with preverbal behavior. It's most effectively conducted through an interactive dialogue, and because it's fairly detailed and lengthy, it can easily fill most of a session. The following dialogue illustrates how the exercise might play out in session.

Therapist: Have you ever had direct experience of a mother cat having a litter of kittens?

Client: Yes.

Therapist: Great! So you may have noticed that when a cat is expecting, the humans around her often prepare a box lined with comfy old towels, which they set in an out-of-the way place, say in a closet. Now imagine that a mother cat has five kittens, conveniently named Kitten Number One, Kitten Number Two, Kitten Number Three, Kitten Number Four, and Kitten Number Five. At first they don't do much. They stay in the box, where they nurse and sleep and their mother cleans them. After their eyes open, they start exploring, and when they do, Kitten Number Five always explores a bit farther than the other kittens and comes back a bit later.

First they explore the box and then come back to nursing. Then they explore the room and come back to nursing. Next they start exploring other rooms, beyond mother cat's line of sight. Throughout, Kitten Number Five always goes a bit farther and returns a bit later. Then, one day, four of the kittens have returned and are nursing, but not Kitten Number Five. He remains somewhere beyond the mother cat's line of sight. Suddenly, she hears the mewling of a kitten in distress. What do we see her do?

Client: Go toward the kitten?

Therapist: Right. By what path?

Client: The shortest?

Therapist:	Exactly. And once she gets to Kitten Number Five, what do we see her do?
Client:	Pick him up by the scruff of his neck and bring him back to the box.
Therapist:	Yes. And what do we see her do next?
Client:	Drop him.
Therapist:	And then?
Client:	Lick him?
Therapist:	Right! Lick him until what?
Client:	Until he's calmed down and gone back to nursing?
Therapist:	Exactly. That's what we see cats do. You know, I don't think only cats do that. In some way or another, we see almost all mammals do that. Except, maybe…
Client:	Humans?
Therapist:	Humans, right! We might see humans do something similar to what cats do: take the shortest path to go meet the little one in distress, bring it to a place of safety, and provide comfort until such time as it's soothed. And you might also see humans do other things.
Client:	Right.
Therapist:	Perhaps we don't always take the shortest path to find our little one who's in danger. In fact, we might say, "Not now, I'm busy. Wait until your father comes back!" Possible or impossible?
Client:	Possible.
Therapist:	Or we might go straight to our little one in distress but then demand an immediate and detailed explanation. Possible or impossible?
Client:	Possible.
Therapist:	Or we might mock: "Look at our courageous explorer—not so courageous anymore!" Possible or impossible?
Client:	Possible.
Therapist:	Or we might invalidate: "Stop whining! You have no reason to be scared!" Possible or impossible?
Client:	Possible.
Therapist:	Or we might threaten: "Stop crying right now, or I'll give you a good reason to cry!" Possible or impossible?

Step 5: Training Self-Compassion   115

Client:	Possible.
Therapist:	Or we might run in the other direction. Possible or impossible?
Client:	Possible.
Therapist:	Or we might cover our ears and say, "I don't want to hear you anymore!" Possible or impossible?
Client:	Possible.
Therapist:	Or we might say, "What did I do to deserve you and all the trouble you cause?" Possible or impossible?
Client:	Possible.
Therapist:	Or we might even roll our eyes and wail, "If only I didn't have you, my life would be so much simpler!" Possible or impossible?
Client:	Possible.
Therapist:	Right. There's a whole range of things that humans can be seen doing other than that instinctive move of going straight to our little one in distress, bringing it to a place of safety, and giving it comfort until it's soothed. And what about you? When Kitten Number Five of your negative self-judgments, shame, or painful feelings or thoughts starts voicing its distress in the distance, what do you notice yourself doing? Do you go straight to it to bring it to a place of safety? Do you comfort it until it's soothed? Or do you notice that you do one of these other things we've just looked at—or perhaps something else?
Client:	(Chuckles.) I sure don't go meet it.
Therapist:	One last thing about Kitten Number Five: Is a kitten in distress more likely to purr or more likely to hiss, spit, scratch, and claw?
Client:	Hiss, spit, and claw.
Therapist:	Right. Okay, now bring to mind something you really don't like about yourself, maybe some painful judgment, feeling, or memory, or something about you or what you do or did that makes you feel ashamed—anything you really don't like when it shows up. See if you can do that. You can either tell me what it is or simply notice it and not tell me what it is. It's your choice.
Client:	I'd rather not say.
Therapist:	That's fine. What's important is that you're able to contact one of your little kittens. Are you?

Client:	Yes.
Therapist:	Great. So, when that little kitten starts hissing and spitting at you, what do you notice yourself doing?
Client:	(*Pauses.*) Actually, I think I scream at it and then try to drown it.
Therapist:	Hmm... And how does it respond to that?
Client:	It hisses, spits, and gets even more aggressive.
Therapist:	So what do you do?
Client:	It depends. Sometimes I try to run away from it. Sometimes I just try to ignore it.
Therapist:	Hmm... How old is that kitten?
Client:	Wow! Real old.
Therapist:	Okay. And what if you asked that kitten what it needs, what would she say?
Client:	I don't know.
Therapist:	Will you ask her?
Client:	Okay. Hmm... Patience and kindness.
Therapist:	Patience and kindness... And how would the mother cat you want to be receive this kitten when she's in distress?
Client:	With patience and kindness. She would go get it and lick it.
Therapist:	Okay, so the mother cat you want to be would go meet it with patience and kindness, and even lick it. Before we next meet, if any of your kittens show up in distress, would you be willing to see if you can notice how you receive them? Do you think you could do that?

In this exchange, the client, who was dealing with some deep-seated shame issues around childhood sexual abuse, chose to not name what her kitten was. That's perfectly okay. In fact, we chose this dialogue in the service of illustrating that this work doesn't depend on content and can be done just as effectively when the therapist doesn't know what the client is contacting. Many clients, however, will be willing to share their kittens, and that's perfectly fine too. In many situations, you may wish to invite clients to have a discussion about their most difficult kittens. In those cases, you can in turn share some of yours, as this may provide high-level validation for your client.

Using an animal metaphor helps distance clients from the verbal rules they may apply to how human children should be treated. It also helps clients connect to more instinctive, preverbal behavior. In our experience, most clients resonate with this metaphor and respond well to the home practice offered at the end of the preceding dialogue. If the client responds well to the kitten image, continue exploring with a few more inquiries into how she relates to the kittens of her distress.

Broadening the Metaphor

If work with this metaphor is going well, extend the discussion using the metaphor to explore some of the deeper implications of turning away from or even against a part of ourselves.

Therapist: I mentioned earlier how it's possible for humans to greet the distress of their little ones by saying, "If only I didn't have you, my life would be so much simpler." Remember?

Client: Yes.

Therapist: Have you ever noticed your mind telling you how much better your life would be if you didn't have that little kitten—that thing you don't like to feel, think, or remember, that harsh self-judgment?

Client: (Chuckles.) Many times!

Therapist: I imagine that if Kitten Number Five got run over by a truck one day, you'd feel intensely relieved.

Client: Yes, of course.

Therapist: So your mind might say, "Your life is going to be so much easier now that Kitten Number Five is gone!" Do you imagine it's possible that your mind might next start looking at Kitten Number Four more closely, and that it might say something like "Well, of course, it's nowhere near as bad as Kitten Number Five, but to be honest, there is this thing about that kitten that just isn't quite right."

Client: Hmm…

Therapist: And do you think it's possible that a little while after that, your mind may start suggesting that your life would be so much better if only Kitten Number Four were gone?

Client: I guess it's possible.

Therapist: Now imagine that Kitten Number Four also gets hit by a truck. Is it possible that after a period of relief, perhaps shorter than the first time, your mind might start looking at Kitten Number Three? That it might say something like "Sure, it's nothing like those other two kittens, but really, there's this thing about Kitten Number Three…"? And do you think it's possible that it may then start telling you how much better your life would be if *that* kitten too was gone?

Client: (*Chuckles.*) Yes, it's possible.

Therapist: So here's my question: Where does it stop? Is this really the kind of mother cats we want to be? Mother cats without kittens? And all this is done against kittens that need…what again? Patience and kindness? You know, I believe those kittens may well be the parts of us that get hooked.

In our experience, clients respond well to this further exploration of the metaphor. The struggle to rid ourselves of thoughts and feelings that we don't like is a war waged against parts of ourselves that have often been with us from an early age. This is a war that cannot be won. If the enemy is part of oneself, who can win? Who can lose?

Looking at Where We Learned to Receive Our Kittens

When we receive our suffering in a different way than a mother cat would receive one of her kittens in distress, we're probably reproducing what we learned from the adults we grew up around. Perhaps our parents or caregivers didn't move toward our distress or that of others around us. Perhaps they didn't meet our missteps with equanimity, a gentle invitation to notice what might have not worked, and warm encouragement to try again at some other time and perhaps in some other way.

After elaborating the metaphor, ask clients whether they might be able to identify whose voice their mind speaks with when they receive their kittens in a way different from how a mother cat would. Alternatively, you can simply invite them to guess who they might have learned this attitude from. Most people model how they receive their distress and missteps on their learning history—their childhood experience of how their own distress and missteps, or those of others, were received. One caution: Be explicit that this work isn't about blame, as it's highly likely that our models in turn based their behavior on the models they grew up with. In fact, what other than getting hooked can lead us to receive little ones in distress with anything other than protection, love, and soothing?

Step 5 Home Practice: Noticing How the Mother Cat Treats Her Kittens

As always, the main home practice exercise is noticing away moves and toward moves. And given that clients to whom you offer the Mother Cat Exercise probably have difficulties with verbal aikido, it may also be a good idea to invite them to continue practicing the verbal aikido moves. Finally, invite them to notice whether any of the kittens of their distress start mewling and hissing, and if they do, how they receive those kittens.

How to Notice and Flexibly Sidestep Potential Traps

In this section, we look in more detail at the potential traps therapists may encounter when training self-compassion in the way outlined in this chapter. In our experience, the Mother Cat Exercise can be highly evocative for clients. They often visibly soften as they start extending more empathy and compassion to the parts of themselves they dislike. For therapists, this exercise is fairly straightforward, so there are only a couple of traps to be mindful of.

Prescribing Compassion as a Rule

Once you understand and truly feel how important self-compassion can be in helping people get unstuck, you may verge on prescribing self-compassion as a rule for clients to follow. And if a given client responds well to new rules, this may appear to work. Unfortunately, this might also undermine clients' psychological flexibility, as all rigid rules can. Plus, if clients find it difficult to take a self-compassionate stance, it's likely that they already live under the yoke of rigid verbal rules that tend to preclude self-compassion. In that case, trying to turn self-compassion into a rigid rule will likely result in increased harsh judgments.

We've found that inviting clients to notice, in session, how they receive their kittens goes a long way toward helping them notice moments when they become harsh with themselves. Similarly, asking how the mother cat they want to be would receive a particular kitten can create enough space for them to notice a broader range of ways to receive their inner experience, beyond their typically harsh and invalidating stance. So practice promoting noticing rather than prescribing rules, no matter how self-compassionate the rule, and see if you notice how deeply healing effective noticing can be.

Dropping the Kittens

It can be particularly painful and distressing to witness clients getting hooked by harsh self-judgments. In some cases, those self-judgments have arisen from horrific trauma or abuse histories, in which case clients may carry an enormous burden of guilt for circumstances in which they were actually hapless victims. It's only human to feel pulled into reassuring such clients or insisting that they aren't at fault. When this happens, you may feel tempted to drop the kitten imagery and start talking about the content of what clients are sharing, if only to express your care.

See if you can resist validating by entering into the content. Instead, validate more broadly with compassionate words, such as "I can see this is really painful for you," and stick with the kittens language. A large part of the power of this metaphor comes from the fact that it cuts through the verbal soup. To see how this works, let's say you drop the kitten talk and start asking a client about how she receives her guilt. She may answer, "With shame. I caused it to happen." Then the conversation could easily veer into a discussion of the client's content and whether she truly was at fault or whether it's appropriate to feel shame. On the other hand, asking with the gentlest compassion, "And how do you receive *that* kitten?" may help the client better notice her relationship with her experience of guilt. This will widen her perspective, rather than narrowing it to a discussion of whether she has good grounds for feeling guilty.

Frequently Asked Questions

What if a client doesn't like cats?

It may be a good idea to ask clients what their favorite animal is or whether they are allergic to or dislike any common pet animals. If a client hates cats, you could go for a mother dog. In an earlier incarnation, this metaphor used a cuddly polar bear mom versus an angry grizzly. But some of our clients could never envision bears as being anything other than vicious, so we settled on a mother cat and her kittens. Cats and dogs are probably the best choices, as most people have direct experience with them. If a client says she loves snakes or some such, do steer her toward mammals, as reptiles and many other nonmammal species often don't display instinctive nurturing behavior.

What if a client's kitten is something awful that I can't in good conscience help her receive kindly?

We heard this question when we were training clinicians working with sexual aggressors. Working with populations whose behaviors significantly deviate from the norm and, just as importantly, go against our own values (for example, pedophiles) presents particular challenges. In this case, it's especially important to frame the kittens as parts of the self the client hates. Then, when drawing out the mother cat's potential behaviors in regard to that kitten, be sure to include submitting to what the kitten demands. The following dialogue illustrates such a situation.

Client:	I guess one of my worst kittens is my urge to watch child pornography.
Therapist:	That's a tough one. Let's look at that kitten of your urge to watch underage porn. When it starts making distress sounds, hissing and spitting at you, how do you receive it?
Client:	I try to ignore it or distract myself. I try to resist it.
Therapist:	Of course you try to resist it. I hope you'll bear with me for a minute as I ask you what may seem like a really strange question. And how does resisting it make that kitten feel?
Client:	I don't know… Worse, I guess. Sometimes it works, and sometimes it just won't shut up, and then…

Therapist:	Yes. Is it okay if I continue with the strange questions?
Client:	Sure.
Therapist:	Are you able to contact that little kitten of your urge to watch child pornography right now?
Client:	Yes.
Therapist:	Okay, so see if you can ask it what it needs—beyond watching porn. Does it have any other needs?
Client:	It needs to leave me alone!
Therapist:	I didn't mean what it needs from your perspective, but from its own perspective. Let me try this: On a line of needing to be rejected here *(opening arms wide and moving left hand)* and being soothed here *(waving right hand)*, where would its needs, from its own perspective, fall?
Client:	I guess more over there *(pointing to therapist's right hand)*.
Therapist:	Wow. And how does the kitten feel, hearing you say that?
Client:	Strange. Quieter, I guess.
Therapist:	That was one courageous piece of work. Over the next week, see if you can notice how you receive that kitten if it starts wailing again.
Client:	Okay.
Therapist:	Before we finish with this, I'd like to ask one thing: How was that whole exchange for you?
Client:	Really strange. You know, I've never ever thought of my urges in that way.
Therapist:	Good. Weird as that may sound, maybe you've milked all you could out of responding to that kitten in a harsh way. I hope you notice some interesting things between now and our next session.

Going Deeper

As we look under the hood to explore some of the processes at work in training self-compassion, we'll dive especially deeply into pliance, the inner rule-giver, and working with rules. This section is somewhat long because it includes a discussion of our vision of how we humans come to hate parts of ourselves and receive them from a less than compassionate stance. For a fuller discussion of compassion as it relates to ACT, we refer you to *The ACT Practitioner's Guide to the Science of Compassion* (Tirch et al., 2014).

Birth of the Inner Rule-Giver

Relative to other mammals, humans display some highly unusual ways of receiving their little ones' distress and missteps. There's a good chance that these behaviors are rooted in what is specific to humans: our ability to talk and think in words.

As children learn to use language and then enter the community of speaking humans, two things happen: they develop the ability to follow increasingly detailed instructions or rules, and then they notice an inner voice speaking to them much as the people around them do. Let's take a peek at what may shape the way this inner voice, which so rarely shuts up, speaks to us.

When you were born, you didn't respond to instructions or rules, only to five-senses experience. Genetically, you were wired to seek food, warmth, and closeness and attention from your caregivers. These hardwired behaviors gave you the best shot at survival in what could otherwise have been a scary and short existence. As you interacted with caregivers and the instructions they gave you, you gradually developed the ability to follow these rules, initially in the form of pliance. As discussed in chapter 2, pliance arises from being directly reinforced for following a rule by whomever proffers the rule.

Ideally, you received positive reinforcement for pliantly following rules, gaining access to reinforcers dispensed by the rule giver. For example, if you shared your toys when instructed to do so, you probably received a hug or praise for being a generous child. The hug or praise added an appetitive consequence, increasing the chances that you would follow the rule again in the future. Such pliance is under appetitive control.

Yet some of the early rules you learned may have taught you to engage in away moves. Maybe a caregiver told you not to approach the hot stove and raised his voice until you started moving away from the stove. This would lead to pliance under aversive control, meaning you followed these rules to move away from unwanted experience delivered by the rule giver, in this case a caregiver scolding you. With pliance under aversive control, reinforcement is negative in the sense that following the rule results in removing, or moving away from, something aversive.

After following rules pliantly, you probably learned to track rules, noticing and being reinforced by consequences beyond receiving approval or avoiding chastisement by rule givers. Such tracking encourages children to contact broader aspects of their experience and consequences beyond those delivered by rule givers. In other words, it promotes noticing. Consider the example of being encouraged to share your toys. Initially, you might have followed this rule pliantly, with the appetitive consequence of receiving praise from a caregiver. However, you might also have been encouraged to notice that when you shared your toys, your playmates looked happier, that they in turn shared their toys and played with you, and that you had a lot of fun together; this would be a cue to engage in tracking. Tracking rules makes for richer conversations and vocabulary as caregivers describe possible consequences the child may notice, whereas demands for pliance make for short conversations that rarely go beyond "because I said so," "because it would make me happy" or "because that's what good kids do."

Soon after children develop the ability to respond pliantly to rules, they are able to produce rules themselves, generally leading to a short period during which they produce rules overtly, pronouncing them to the world. Then they stop proffering every rule loudly and the inner rule-giver gets going. (Of course, there isn't an actual inner rule-giver; rather, we engage in rule-forming behavior, the products of which can occasion and consequate behavior.) With the onset of this inner rule-forming behavior, your mind started talking to you, and if it's anything like ours, it probably hasn't shut up for a second since that day. The productions of that inner rule-forming behavior may well be a function of the early rule-giving contexts you were exposed to. If early in your verbal development you were exposed to a high ratio of contexts in which pliance was reinforced over tracking, you may notice your inner rule-giver pulling for pliance over tracking. With clients, this may take the form of saying that they're just "like this" or that they behaved a certain way because they have to or because they've always done so.

It's also worthwhile to pay attention to whether inner rules tend to be under appetitive or aversive control. If early pliance was largely under aversive control, this may turn the inner rule-giver into an aversive-control freak that produces a plethora of rules along the lines of "You mustn't do this," "Don't do this or you'll be punished," "If you do this, it means you're a loser," and so on.

Similarly, if your early experience with tracking rules was largely under aversive control ("Don't do this or you won't get that" or "If you do that, this list of bad outcomes will follow"), you may find that your inner rule-giver sounds like a raging worrywart. This can cause rules to be tracked in unworkable and avoidant ways, especially when they're negatively reinforced. People may come to respond pliantly, counterpliantly, or with avoidant tracking. The latter, avoidant tracking, can be highly tricky, as "noticing" that, as a result of avoidance, any number of imagined bad outcomes don't occur (as they often don't) can reinforce avoidant tracking and feed worry.

Tracking can also become a problem when it's narrow and restricted to a few aspects of the context, and particularly when only short-term consequences are tracked. For example, consider someone who's prone to social anxiety. She may track that by not going to parties, she doesn't feel social anxiety, rather than tracking that, in the long term, she doesn't make friends or expand her network, which may be important to her. At its most extreme, both inner and outer rule-giving may become so aversive that people move away from most rule-giving contexts, including the well-intentioned ACT-congruent rules you may offer in the context of therapy. People with such responses to rule giving can be among the most difficult clients.

We believe that the way people receive the kittens of their distress and negative self-judgments has a lot to do with the early rule-giving contexts they were exposed to. Our inner rule-giving behavior may pick up caregivers' dominant modes of responding to distress and missteps and produce its own mix of pliance and tracking. When these are largely under aversive control, harsh self-judgments and fear of inner experience are dominant and may impede therapeutic progress. This is why we believe it can be useful to pay attention to pliance, to tracking that's largely limited to controlling inner experience, and, more generally, to rule-governed behavior under aversive control.

Using Rules in Clinical Practice

Rules are useful. They allow us to navigate life without needing to experience everything firsthand before deciding what to move toward and away from, much like using a GPS to find our way in an unfamiliar city. The most useful rules are those that promote tracking. However, it's important to promote tracking that's sensitive to the broadest aspects of the context and to both short-term and long-term consequences of behavior.

Keeping an eye out for both pliance and tracking in clients can make interventions more powerful. If you feel that pliance or counterpliance may be evoked, gently alert your client to the possibility that her mind might try to turn whatever you said into a rigid rule, whereas you're only inviting her to notice what shows up. Once a client has derived rigid rules—whether she couches them in terms of what she must do or in terms of what she must do to be a good client—it will likely keep her stuck in away moves: moving away from either disobeying (pliance) or obeying (counterpliance). Assure your client that this is normal and that there is another way: simply noticing what's happening and sorting it onto the matrix. When you do this, you invite clients to practice flexible tracking, noticing broad consequences and aspects of their experience beyond what their minds tell them that they should do or that you want them to do, or about how things should be.

Keeping an eye out for aversive and appetitive control is also useful and can enhance clinical interventions. Use as much appetitive control as you possibly can. To that end, refrain from delivering aversive consequences, such as expressing negative judgments that may arise when clients don't do their home practice exercises or when they continue to engage in the behaviors that feed their stuck loops. On the tracking side, go easy on inviting clients to notice the aversive consequences of their behavior. For example, if you ask clients whether an away behavior takes them toward or away from who or what is important when it's clear that it moves them away, you risk making such questions, and eventually yourself, aversive. In other words, you risk having clients conflate the matrix, yourself, and therapy as a whole with a judging parent—not a good place from which to effectively train flexibility!

Clients who tend to follow rules in a mostly pliant manner will naturally look for rules to respond to pliantly everywhere. Their minds will try to seize anything you say and turn it into a rule they can follow pliantly. In such cases, although outwardly it may look as though they are getting it and making progress, they're actually just doing more of the same. With these clients, we seek to create contexts for flexible tracking to train them to pay attention to aspects of their experience that go beyond pliance or avoidant tracking. This is where pointing rather than telling comes into its own. The basic verbal aikido moves, and matrix work in general, can have such a function because, in all situations, clients are encouraged to sort and track the different aspects of their experience. The matrix practitioner seeks mostly to point toward experience rather than pull for particular content or behavior—other than the behavior of noticing what experience may lie in the direction we point toward. Don't hesitate to be explicit about this by telling clients that you can only point, and only they can notice because only they experience what they are experiencing. Mention that because of this, your words count for very little and their noticing for everything.

One final note on pliance and tracking: These are not ways of speaking, but ways in which people interact with rules. They are functions. The best way to work with them is to practice noticing the difference in how they feel and then invite clients to notice how things are working for them.

In the Frame

In terms of derived relational responding, the Mother Cat Exercise and other such approaches can have a powerful effect in transforming the functions of intensely aversive inner stimuli. Harsh self-judgments are notoriously difficult to change, and when people are profoundly hooked, they tend to resort to away moves and find themselves in stuck loops. When the Mother Cat Exercise works, the texture of these parts of a person's experiences and self-judgments might shift from rough and aversive to softer, more appetitive functions. You can verify this after the exercise by asking clients to evaluate whether they feel more inclined to approach the kittens of their distress, rather than moving away from them.

Framing can also be a powerful influence in shaping rules and rule-governed behavior. We can frame things in such a way as to make a particular action more or less probable somewhat independently of the five-senses consequences that may follow. Maybe Dad says to three-year-old Timmy, "Only big boys of four are able to help empty the dishwasher," and notices that Timmy insists on helping him empty the dishwasher, whereas if he had just said, "Timmy, would you help me empty the dishwasher?" he might have noticed Timmy making a beeline for his toy truck. The consequences of emptying the dishwasher remain the same: Dad giving Timmy a hug and saying, "You've helped me empty the dishwasher. You're such a sweet boy!" Yet framing emptying the dishwasher with "big boys of four" could increase the reinforcing power of Dad's invitation if being a bigger boy is appetitive to Timmy and Timmy himself put the augmental into action by telling himself that big boys help with the dishwasher. Such framing serves as an augmental, increasing the probability of the behavior, as discussed in chapter 4. This is the power of derived relational responding.

This form of rule-following behavior is known as augmenting. It's a particular verbal process wherein framing things in a certain way changes the reinforcing properties of a given behavior or makes some other reinforcer that's less accessible more salient and valuable. Augmenting can make moving toward more attractive or make moving away more aversive. Advertising works through augmenting. For example, a brand of soda may sponsor a basketball player. Nothing changes in the world of five-senses experience, but if you admire that player, that particular brand of soda may become a bit more attractive to you as you tell yourself that you're drinking your hero's favorite soft drink.

Augmenting can be done under appetitive control. For example, let's say you put a motivational poster titled "Winners" on your wall. It has an inspiring photograph, and underneath it is the caption "Never give up." Now imagine that while surfing the Internet you see another poster with a similarly inspiring photograph and the selfsame title: "Winners." But the caption on this one reads, "Because nothing says 'Loser' more than a motivational poster about winners." You may instantly decide to take your poster down. Notice that nothing has changed in the world of five-senses experience. The only change was in the kind of self-rule generated by seeing the poster: you started telling yourself, "Losers need posters." So when seeking to cue augmenting, keep an eye out for augmenting under aversive control versus augmenting under appetitive control and aim for the latter, just as when working with pliance or tracking.

We find that augmenting is a powerful tool that can help clients more easily choose moving toward who or what is important to them. In some ACT books, you may find exercises that advocate using augmenting to motivate people to move away from the aversive consequences of their stuck behaviors. An example would be inviting clients to contemplate where they'll find themselves in ten years' time if they keep doing things in the same way. We aren't convinced augmenting under aversive control is an optimal strategy for getting people unstuck. In our experience, deliberately creating an appetitive learning context is a highly effective way to help clients get unstuck fast. Further, we've found that augmenting works best when accomplished through broad, open questions that allow clients to derive their own appetitive functions for choices that they're unable to make when they're stuck. As mentioned in chapter 4, an extremely powerful question for this purpose is "What would the person you want to be do?" In our experience, people who are stuck tend to be sensitive to aversive control and react to it by digging in all the more. Therefore, we choose our words carefully so we don't appear to be trying to lead them to a predetermined place, which could give rise to pliant or counterpliant responses.

Here again, early learning history probably plays a large role in how our minds use augmentals. For example, if someone has been teased and mocked a lot or judged as defective, it's likely that her mind will produce augmentals based on aversive control. If this were the case for a client with panic attacks, she might experience her mind telling her that only losers fear panic sensations. Though this might make it aversive for her to engage in avoidance under the control of fear, it's more likely to keep her in stuck loops where moving away from being a loser competes with moving away from the fear of panic. In that competition, the likely winner is the more habitual behavior of moving away from the fear of panic. And even if she does stop avoiding in order to move away from acting like a loser, this wouldn't bring a sense of vitality, so the client would probably feel as stuck as ever.

This is the dark side of augmenting: it can keep people stuck. An augmental such as "Good people don't feel anxiety," for example, can increase the likelihood of away moves in the presence of anxiety. In such cases, bringing the spotlight back to overt behavior can be a great help. A question such as "What would the person you want to be do in a situation like this?" can go a long way toward weakening problematic augmentals. Just be sure to frame this question in terms of observable behavior (what the client would like to do), rather than thoughts or feelings.

When in doubt about the effects of augmentals—yours or your client's—share your concern and ask the client whether what you or she just said would make her more likely to choose a toward or an away move.

Promoting Flexible Tracking Through the Matrix

The quadrants and discriminations of the matrix are powerful cues that encourage tracking. The vertical line cues clients to track both their inner experience and their outer, five-senses context. The horizontal line cues them to track the function of their behaviors—whether they are toward or away moves. Depending on the context, function can be tracked in a number of ways. Early in your work with a given client, it may be most effective to concentrate on toward and away from aspects of experience based in verbal functions (toward who or what is important versus away from unwanted inner stuff). Later, you may find it more effective to help clients track whether their behavior takes them toward or away from five-senses experience, from particular feelings (as in the case of sensation seeking), or from who or what is important, all of which can serve to make toward behavior more appetitive and help clients sort between workable and unworkable away moves.

The practitioner's aim is to constantly orient toward flexible tracking while subtly undermining excessive pliance. You can do this in a number of ways—for example, through the routine around telling clients they don't have to do the home practice exercises. Naming the possibility of pliance (though we don't recommend you use the word with clients) whenever this could be showing up is another move that makes it easier for clients to track some of the consequences of their pliance—for example, making you feel that the client is engaged when she's really just following orders.

Step 5 Checklist

Use this checklist (available for download at http://www.newharbinger.com/33605) to guide your practice of the strategies outlined in this chapter.

What I did

☐ I checked with my client about how her verbal aikido practice was going and invited her to engage in a couple of rounds of verbal aikido using situations of her choice.

☐ I presented the Mother Cat Exercise in the form of a dialogue.

☐ I made sure to keep my client engaged by asking her if the human behaviors I described were possible or impossible.

☐ I invited my client to contact at least one negative self-judgment, highly distressing emotion or sensation, or part of herself she hates and then referred to it as a kitten in distress.

☐ I asked my client to notice how she receives that kitten when it starts mewling in the distance.

☐ I asked my client how the mother cat she wants to be would receive that particular kitten in distress.

☐ I asked my client to ask her kitten what it needed.

☐ I asked my client about her experience of practicing this exercise.

☐ I invited my client to notice how she receives the kittens of her distress over the coming days.

What I didn't overdo

☐ Getting hooked by the content of what my client presented as her kitten and getting pulled into a discussion of that content

☐ Dropping the kitten talk and referring to my client's negative self-judgment, distress, or other hated part of herself as a self-judgment, distress, or part of herself

☐ Giving my client instructions about how to receive her kittens

☐ Letting my client speak for her kitten from the perspective of what her mind tells her the kitten needs, rather than from the perspective of the kitten's needs

CHAPTER 6

Step 6: Harnessing the Power of Perspective Taking

Once clients are able to practice the basic verbal aikido moves and recognize how they receive the kittens of their harsh self-judgments, they may still need a gentle nudge to make good on the promise to more easily choose to engage in toward moves even in the presence of what they don't want to think or feel. Some clients may say they understand everything yet still stay stuck.

Step 6 seeks to address this difficulty by harnessing the power of perspective taking, a process that lies at the core of the matrix, and of ACT more generally. In this chapter, we'll guide you through a powerful perspective-taking exercise that can help clients get unstuck fast. We'll also explore why perspective-taking is so central to ACT and the matrix approach. Of course, this exercise can also benefit clients who aren't profoundly stuck. Indeed, it can help anyone develop a greater ability to choose to engage in values-congruent action, even in the presence of significant inner obstacles.

Opening the Session

As with previous sessions, you can begin with the brief settling-in exercise. Next, debrief the home practice: noticing toward and away moves and whether clients noticed any kittens and how they received them. This will give you a good feel for how clients have progressed in developing more psychological flexibility. As the Mother Cat Exercise does its work, you'll notice clients becoming visibly kinder to themselves. As an example, the week after we conducted the exercise with a teenager living with anorexia, at the beginning of her next session she reported that noticing her harsh body-image self-judgments and rigid dietary rules as kittens had helped her significantly increase her food intake. In fact, her doctor could hardly believe how much weight she'd put on in just one week.

Conducting the Perspective-Taking Interview

The majority of this session is devoted to an interview that deliberately activates perspective taking in the service of helping clients get unstuck in targeted situations. It involves asking clients to choose a situation in the near future in which they anticipate getting stuck and then inviting them to engage in a dialogue between their here-now and there-then perspectives. It's an effective way of promoting psychological flexibility, especially if you guide clients in shifting perspectives numerous times. After doing this exercise, clients often notice that they can more readily choose to engage in a toward move when the anticipated situation arises.

Note that this aspect of the exercise also makes it an excellent evaluation tool. In our experience, clients who can easily shift perspectives during the interview tend to be most likely to engage in the dialogue when they next find themselves in the stuck situation, and they often notice getting unstuck as a result.

The broad outlines of the interview are as follows:

1. Help clients choose a near-future situation in which they anticipate getting stuck in an away move when engaging in a toward move would be important. The chosen situation should be anticipated to occur at a definite time and place and have a high probability of coming up before your next therapy session.

2. "Teleport" clients to meet themselves in that situation when it next arises and invite them to engage in a present-tense dialogue between their here-now and there-then perspectives. In this exchange, you'll play the role of an impartial journalist, making sure each perspective speaks in turn and regularly checking in with your here-now client to see how the there-then perspective receives what the here-now client says. You may at times need to intervene (with permission) to invite the here-now perspective to validate the there-then perspective by acknowledging how hard it is to be stuck.

3. When you notice a shift toward increased flexibility in the dialogue, facilitate a few more changes in perspective. Then have the client ask what, specifically, the there-then perspective will do in the target situation.

4. Finally, you'll debrief the interview, asking clients how the exchange felt and whether they noticed any changes over the course of the dialogue. Then ask how likely they feel it is that they will indeed engage in a similar exchange in the target situation. Invite them to let you know by e-mail or text message what they noticed when the anticipated situation arose. (Clients can also inform you about this using the Matrix Session Bridging Questionnaire, which we provide in chapter 7.)

The form and content of the interview should themselves be flexible and chosen to meet the needs of individual clients. Therefore, we'll present the interview via an example dialogue. The client is Julia, a thirty-two-year-old who has been besieged by obsessions centered on the possibility that her kitchen appliances may catch fire.

Therapist: We've gone through a lot of what I want to show you, and you've made amazing progress. Today I thought it might be helpful to see what else we can do to help you get unstuck in future situations. Can you imagine yourself getting stuck over the next few days? In other words, do you anticipate any situations in which you might get hooked into away moves, despite wanting to engage in toward moves?

Client: Sure, tonight!

Therapist: Cool. Where will you be?

Client: In my kitchen.

Therapist: When?

Client: Bedtime. Around ten o'clock.

Therapist: Can you picture what you'll see around you?

Client: Sure. There's the kitchen counter, the sink, the walls, the dishwasher, the stove, the oven…

Therapist: Excellent. Are you there now?

Client: Yes.

Therapist: Okay, now imagine that I could teleport you-here-now to go meet Julia in her kitchen at ten o'clock tonight.

Client: Okay…

Therapist: Okay, so you're now there with Julia. Is there something you can tell Julia that may be helpful to her? From now on, I'll ask you to speak to Julia directly—in the present tense. After all, you are both present in the kitchen.

Client: I could say…

Therapist: (Interrupts.) Don't use "coulds." You're there with her. Just go ahead and speak to Julia.

Client: "Stop checking! You know it's useless."

Therapist: Great! And how does Julia receive what you just told her?

Client: Not well.

Therapist: Oh, right. What does she say in response?

Client: She says, "Leave me alone!"

Therapist: Okay. Is there anything else you can tell Julia?

Step 6: Harnessing the Power of Perspective Taking   133

Client:	I could…
Therapist:	Remember, no "coulds." Just go ahead and say it.
Client:	"You know that checking will only get you more stuck."
Therapist:	And how does Julia take that?
Client:	She says, "I know!"
Therapist:	How does Julia feel?
Client:	She's pissed.
Therapist:	Ask Julia what tone of voice you're speaking to her in.
Client:	She says it's kind of sharp.
Therapist:	What tone does Julia need to be spoken to in?
Client:	A kinder tone, I guess.
Therapist:	Want to try it?
Client:	"Julia, you know this won't help."
Therapist:	How did Julia take that?
Client:	A bit better.
Therapist:	Is there anything else you want to say to Julia?
Client:	I don't know what else I could say.
Therapist:	Would you like me to suggest something?
Client:	Sure.
Therapist:	Try telling Julia something like "It's hard" or "I know it's hard."
Client:	"Julia, I know it's hard."
Therapist:	How does Julia receive that?
Client:	(*Starts tearing up.*) She says, "Yes, it's hard."
Therapist:	Did that work better?
Client:	Yes.
Therapist:	Is there anything else you'd like to tell Julia?

Client:	"I know, Julia. I'm there for you."
Therapist:	How does Julia receive that?
Client:	She feels heard.
Therapist:	Great! What do you see Julia do next?
Client:	She checks one last time and goes to the bedroom to spend time with her boyfriend.
Therapist:	Excellent. Is there one last thing you'd like to tell Julia before you come back to the here and now?
Client:	*(Tears up again.)* Yes. "Julia, I'm going to be there for you."
Therapist:	Wow. How did Julia take that?
Client:	She's grateful and she feels less alone.
Therapist:	Great work. Let's return to the here and now. *(Pauses.)* So, how was it for you to be teleported to your kitchen tonight and meet Julia there?
Client:	It was weird—and hard.
Therapist:	Did you notice anything happening?
Client:	*(Giggles.)* Sure. I noticed I got softer as time went on.
Therapist:	Did that work for Julia?
Client:	Oh yes. That's just what she needed.
Therapist:	Isn't it interesting how we speak to ourselves when we get stuck?
Client:	Hmm…
Therapist:	I say "we" because I can easily catch myself doing it too.
Client:	Really?
Therapist:	Sure. Now tell me: How would you rate the probability that you'll actually go and meet Julia in her kitchen tonight and have this kind of a dialogue with her?
Client:	Maybe 90 percent.
Therapist:	That's interesting. Will you text me to let me know what you notice?
Client:	Sure.

Step 6: Harnessing the Power of Perspective Taking

Julia did text her therapist that night. She had noticed that she had a dialogue somewhat similar to the one conducted in session. The way she described it was that she noticed herself speaking more kindly to herself, in particular telling herself how hard it was to be stuck there. In her next session, she commented on how unusual and powerful that approach had been. She said she had noticed that she let go of checking and went to join her boyfriend in the bedroom. And she jokingly commented that her boyfriend had approved of her choosing that particular toward move over another thirty minutes of checking her kitchen appliances. Julia also reported that she started noticing that she spoke to herself in kinder ways when she got stuck. From that time on, her compulsions started diminishing significantly, as she noticed herself engaging in more toward moves in situations where, in the past, she would have engaged in her compulsions. A few months later, Julia became pregnant, a dream she had all but abandoned due to the challenges she had faced in being preoccupied with her compulsions.

Debriefing the Exercise

Once you bring the dialogue to a close, be sure to debrief the exercise by asking your here-now client how this dialogue was for him, as the therapist did in the preceding dialogue by asking "So how was it for you to be teleported to your kitchen tonight and meet Julia there?" This is extremely important, as it increases the probability that the client will engage in a similar dialogue when he next finds himself in that stuck situation, and perhaps others, as well.

To debrief, ask your client whether he noticed any moments in the exchange when things shifted for either perspective. Did it feel as though the exchange was getting harder and more stuck? Did it feel as though it was getting softer and more flexible? Did any particular words shift things for either of the client's perspectives? Bring a spirit of open curiosity to this conversation and have your client revisit the dialogue in detail. If you noticed any changes—whether salient or more subtle—offer your observations and see how the client responds. Here, as always, hold your thoughts lightly and demonstrate that you're willing to let go if the client doesn't recognize what you thought you saw. After all, this intervention is about helping your client notice his experience, not about convincing him that the dialogue led to some major change. So be open to whatever shows up, and reinforce all noticing on the client's part.

As a final step in debriefing, ask what estimate your here-now client puts on the probability that he will indeed show up in the stuck situation and have this kind of dialogue with himself. Regardless of the estimate, you can respond with something like "That's interesting. I'm looking forward to hearing what you noticed."

Perspective Taking with Past Hurts

With many clients, we've found it most effective to concentrate on present situations, whether from the recent past (the past week or two) or the near future (the next week or two) when doing this perspective-taking work. When engaging in perspective-taking dialogues, clients often surprise us by finding ways to make room for the parts of their past that reactivate in the present, making it unnecessary to fish out a past situation in which they can comfort a younger self who faced fear, loneliness, trauma, or rejection or who didn't receive the love and validation that younger self needed.

At times, perspective-taking exercises aimed at traumatic or hurtful situations from the past may also prove useful. Translating this approach into matrix terms, you can invite clients to sort a traumatic or hurtful situation from the distant past onto the matrix. Alternatively, you can conduct a perspective-taking dialogue similar to that outlined in this chapter. Some clients who have carried the burden of very painful past traumas have reported that such exercises are both unforgettable and highly effective for getting unstuck.

In practice, we've found that the Mother Cat Exercise, described in chapter 5, can do a lot of this work in a way that bypasses some the language-related problems that can get in the way when the approach centers on verbal humans. Verbal rules about human parenting and what children are supposed to feel and do can be so strong that they may stand in the way of effective past-centered work. Here's a memorable example of what can go wrong when conducting a dialogue with deep past hurts: In the middle of a perspective-taking exercise with herself as a six-year-old child, one of our clients flatly advised her six-year-old self to kill herself. Yet that same client didn't choose to be the kind of mother cat who ignores her kittens, much less drowns them or tells them to run under a bus. Verbal humans tend to bring their entire verbal history with them, and sometimes this gets in the way of effective perspective-taking work.

Home Practice: Meeting Oneself in Future Stuck Situations

The home practice exercise for this step is for clients to notice whether their anticipated stuck situation arises, and if it does, whether they have a dialogue with themselves similar to the one conducted in session. Inviting clients to e-mail or text what they noticed can be a powerful cue for increasing the probability that they'll engage in the dialogue. That said, in our experience the in-session dialogue is memorable enough that clients usually notice using a similar approach in their actual stuck situations.

As for all earlier sessions, you can also invite clients to keep noticing toward and away moves. As this step concludes the six-step matrix approach, the current session might be one of the last times you meet with a given client. So this could also be a good time to clearly establish that getting unstuck is a lifelong practice that involves practicing all the skills explored in the six steps:

- Noticing toward and away moves

- Noticing the effectiveness of away moves in the short term, in the long term, and to help them move toward who or what is important

- Noticing the difference between five-senses and inner or mental experience

- Noticing hooks and what they do next

- Practicing verbal aikido

- Noticing how they receive the kittens of their distress

- Noticing how they talk to themselves in stuck situations

Among these skills, we believe that noticing toward and away moves may subsume all the others, as practicing the skills in stuck situations is likely to serve as a toward move that can be noticed. Further, the cumulative effect of practicing the flexibility skills inherent in the six steps can recalibrate clients' inner compass in such a way that they can notice how it feels to move toward, how it feels to move away, and how it feels to do something to get back to moving toward; then all of this will progressively become more automatic and implicit. As their compass gradually recalibrates, they can then phase out their practice of the more formal and somewhat cognitively taxing exercises, such as verbal aikido. Of course, clients can return to practicing more intentionally any time the going gets tough.

How to Notice and Flexibly Sidestep Potential Traps

The perspective-taking interview is a highly technical skill, and a number of potential traps can arise when conducting it. As you start using the interview with clients, don't be discouraged if you notice yourself falling into some of these traps. Remember that, for you just as for your clients, mistakes are an essential—often even precious—part of learning. Stick with it, and you and your clients will experience the power of this exercise. Also, note that although some of the tips here may seem like a rehash of the recommendations above, they are so important that we want to emphasize them.

Focusing on the Distant Future or Unlikely Situations

Sometimes clients offer a situation in the distant future to use in the interview. Likewise, they may choose situations that are unlikely to occur, whether in the short term or the long term. If you go along with such choices, clients probably won't get a chance to notice the effects of the in-session dialogue, as it's unlikely to remain salient in their awareness over the long term. Furthermore, you won't get a chance to debrief what happened in your next session, so the whole thing risks getting lost in the mist of time. If this happens, gently ask clients whether they'd be willing to focus on one of the stuck situations most likely to come up next. The sooner the situation is likely to arise, the more likely the exercise is to be effective.

Working on Vague Situations

Similarly, clients may offer vague situations as the context for the interview, like "arguing with my spouse." Unfortunately, vague situations lend themselves to vague, generalized dialogues that don't get to the heart of the matter. Think of this as a teleportation exercise. If you don't set a precise spatiotemporal teleportation target, your client is likely to get atomized in some cosmic wormhole. On a more practical level, it will be more difficult for your client to engage in a focused dialogue. As the operator of the teleportation system, it is your responsibility to help the client choose a clear target.

If clients initially offer a vague situation, ask them to zero in on a particular time and place; for example, "arguing with my spouse about whose turn it is to do the laundry, probably tonight." If clients aren't certain when and where they might next get stuck, invite them to just imagine a precise time and place. This precision serves two functions: allowing clients to engage in a very specific dialogue, and increasing the chances that the dialogue will take place in the next stuck situation.

Being Confused and Confusing in Naming the Perspectives

If you refer to the here-now perspective as "you-here-now" and the there-then perspective as "you-there-then," you may notice that both you and your clients quickly get confused about what perspective each refers to. Instead, refer to the client's here-now perspective with "you" and his future perspective using his first name. During the interview, be as consistent as you can in maintaining this distinction. So if a client's name is Manuel, your questions will go something like this: "So how does Manuel receive what you just told him?" "What does Manuel say to you in response?" "What do you say in response to what Manuel just said?" Even so, it may feel confusing at times. Don't worry; with practice you'll get the hang of it.

Getting Lost in Conditionals

Gently coach clients to conduct the dialogue in the present tense. In this exercise, clients tend to readily slip into conditional verbs: "I could say that Manuel knows that won't help," "Manuel would tell me to go screw myself," and so on. When you notice that happening, gently coach clients to address their other perspective directly using the present tense so that in response to your question "What do you say to Manuel?" your client says, speaking directly to there-then Manuel, "You know that won't help." Then, in response to your question "And what does Manuel respond to that?" your here-now client tells you that Manuel says, "Go screw yourself,'" and so on. You can help by resolutely sticking with the present tense yourself. So rather than asking, "What could you tell Manuel that could be helpful?" instead ask, "What can you tell Manuel that could be useful?" To that, you might add, "Once you know, just go ahead and tell

Manuel." If clients slip into conditionals or you feel that they're talking to you rather than to their there-then perspective, gently remind them that they're present with their self in the future and can therefore talk directly in the present tense to their other perspective.

Getting Stuck on One Perspective

In this exercise, flexibility emerges as a function of repeatedly shifting perspectives between here-now and there-then in the next stuck situation. Clients don't need to linger very long in one perspective; indeed, this wouldn't be helpful. So remember to think of your role as being similar to a journalist keeping a television debate alive by giving the microphone to one person and then the next, and not letting any participant hog the mike for long. Help the client shift from the here-now perspective to the there-then perspective as often as you can. As you first practice using this exercise, you might even inwardly count the perspective reversals.

Getting Hooked by Content

Sometimes you may not get what clients are talking about and feel drawn to ask for clarification. Alternatively, you may disagree with clients' self-judgments. In either case, be aware that the content of what clients are saying may hook you. If you notice a pull to ask questions about what clients are saying rather than how they receive and respond to what's being said from both the here-now and there-then perspectives, just notice that hook and see if you can let it go. If you do bite, it's likely that you and the client will get entangled in a discussion that will pull him away from the dialogue.

Intervening Heavily in the Conversation

Essentially, you want this to be a conversation between the client's two perspectives, not a three-way exchange. Intervene as little as possible. Again, your role is more akin to that of a neutral journalist conducting a debate and not contributing much content. To the greatest extent possible, refer to the client's experience—for example, by asking the client to notice how his there-then perspective receives what the here-now client says. For example, you might ask, "And how does Manuel receive what you just told him?"

If you feel you have to intervene in the conversation beyond asking how the there-then perspective receives what the here-now client says and what either replies to the other's words or tone of voice, direct your interventions to the here-now perspective. The reason for this is that the here-now perspective effectively represents the client's inner rule-giver as it shows up in stuck situations. By directing interventions toward this perspective, you're more likely to have an impact.

Validating the There-Then Perspective

When things get tough and clients start crying, you may be tempted to intervene to validate the there-then perspective. However, doing so may diminish the here-now client's motivation or need to provide validation and shortchange him of a learning opportunity. Ultimately, this may reduce the chances that the client can self-validate in his next stuck situation. So instead, see if you can invite the here-now perspective to validate the there-then perspective.

In contrast, you may occasionally need to validate the client's here-now perspective. For example, if the client notices that this exercise is hard to do, validate that the exercise is hard. The most effective validations are usually the simplest, such as "It's hard" or, if you need extra-strength validation, "It's *really* hard." Use simple language that's as close to the client's own language as possible to ensure that the client can receive the proffered validation as his own. If you use convoluted formulations, you run the risk that your client will interact with your words, rather than his experience.

When things seem really sticky and the client's here-now perspective is unable to find validating words, have the here-now client ask the there-then perspective what it needs to hear. Then invite the here-now client to say it. That said, there are times when the there-then perspective won't know. In those cases, the basic validation "It's hard" or the stronger version "It's really hard" will probably work its magic.

Moving Too Fast

This exercise is highly effective as a prompt for behavior change when clients find themselves in stuck situations in the near future. When clients show flexibility in the dialogue, behavior change often follows in subsequent real-life situations. To promote this during the dialogue, once you see signs of flexibility you can ask the client's here-now perspective what the there-then perspective does next. However, do take your time and be careful not to ask too early, as this might lead to a stuck answer.

When you do notice a shift toward greater flexibility in the dialogue, allow clients to shift perspectives a few more times. Then, and only then, ask what the there-then perspective does next. If you ask this question too early in the exchange, the answer is likely to be that the there-then perspective will engage in an away move. If this happens, facilitate the client in continuing with the dialogue and again watch for increased flexibility.

Be aware that such tipping points don't always arise; it can occasionally happen flexibility doesn't show up. In such cases, it's better not to ask what the there-then perspective does next. Just go straight to debriefing the exercise. As a next step, you may need to ask the client for permission to work on a couple of other situations, perhaps choosing easier ones. In some cases, clients won't be able to shift perspectives easily. In that event, you may need to practice perspective taking in a more piecemeal way before returning to this exercise. A great way to do that is by practicing the verbal aikido moves a few more times.

Not Being Prepared for Goofiness

Sometimes these dialogues get emotional, and sometimes they get goofy. Let go of any expectations and be open to whatever may show up. To demonstrate the kind of goofiness that can arise, consider the following example, in which Sonia, who is thirteen years old, had a spirited dialogue with her future self, who was stuck in an argument with her younger sister, Beth, over emptying the dishwasher.

Sonia here-now: Sonia, it's only a stupid plate. Let it go.

Sonia there-then: Who the hell are you? Where are you coming from? Get the hell out of here!

Sonia here-now: Er… I come from your past, Sonia. I am you.

Sonia there-then: That's freaking weird. What do you want?

Sonia here-now: I want to help you. You don't have to fight over this!

Sonia there-then: Easy for you to say. But Beth really gets on my nerves!

Sonia here-now: *(Turns to therapist.)* What should I say?

Therapist: What does Sonia need to hear?

Sonia here-now: Let me ask. *(Pauses.)* She says she needs me to see how irritating Beth is.

Therapist: Okay, can you tell her that?

Sonia here-now: *(Frowns.)* Oh, all right then. Hey, you from the future, I know she's really irritating!

Sonia there-then: Yeah, she freaking is!

When Sonia came to her next session and her therapist asked her what she'd noticed, she responded, "Nothing." When her therapist inquired what she meant by that, she responded that she hadn't had a single fight with her sister around the dishwasher—a fight that had previously occurred on a regular basis.

Frequently Asked Questions

What if clients anticipate that they won't be able to have this dialogue in their future stuck situation?

This isn't a problem. Validate that things may look and feel hard from where they're standing now, and show an interest in whatever they notice when the situation arises.

Similarly, if clients estimate that there's only a very low probability that they can meet their there-then perspective in the stuck situation and engage in such a dialogue, simply express an interest in whatever they notice. In either case, ask them to let you know via an e-mail or text message.

How can I increase the chances that clients will conduct the dialogue when in the situation?

The more salient the situation is to clients, the more likely it is that they'll engage in the dialogue when the real-life situation arises. In addition, we've found it quite effective to ask clients to send us a brief e-mail or text message sharing what they noticed when their targeted stuck situation arose. This serves as a reminder and makes it highly likely that clients will notice themselves getting hooked and then choose to engage in this sort of dialogue with themselves.

How is this different from empty chair work?

At first blush, this exercise may seem so much like empty chair work that you may be tempted to use an empty chair to conduct it. We recommend against doing so, if for no other reason than that clients won't necessarily be sitting when the stuck situation actually arises. That said, feel free to adapt this exercise and notice what shows up.

One crucial way in which this exercise differs from empty chair work is in having a very precise focus. Whereas in empty chair work the dialogue often targets past hurts and difficult relationships, the perspective-taking interview zeros in on the near future and a stuck situation—one in which the client anticipates not being able to engage in a toward move. We've found that this precision in focus allows difficult emotional content to show up in a context in which its behavioral functions are more apparent to the client. By addressing hooks and painful inner experience in this more behaviorally focused context, we promote workability, rather than affective or cognitive change per se.

Further, in this exercise the emphasis is on shifting perspectives as often as possible, which allows empathy and self-compassion to emerge as a function of the client's increased ability to flexibly shift perspective, whereas in empty chair work the emphasis may be on trying to come to some sort of emotional reconciliation. Although this may seem like a subtle distinction, we feel it's a distinction that makes a difference.

Going Deeper

In this chapter, we'll go deeper by exploring values work, as values are central to behavior change in ACT. We'll also look at why perspective taking is essential to psychological flexibility and how it fosters empathy, compassion, and self-compassion while increasing behavior under the appetitive control of values.

Navigating Values Conflicts

Perspective taking is central to dealing with what some clients and many therapists term "values conflicts." It's easy to tie oneself in knots around the phrase "values conflict," and it's not uncommon for the words "values conflict" to appear as a hook. However, when people mention values conflicts, this is an indication that they notice multiple people or things as being important to them. This is a good problem to have! It means they notice a plurality of potential sources of reinforcement.

Doing ACT with the matrix is about helping people take perspective so they can more easily choose to do what's important to them in the presence of obstacles. And when they notice multiple people or things being important to them, they'll eventually notice choosing between them. In some cases, they may notice that choosing the same action is a move toward a number of important people and things. For example, they may choose to take their family for a Sunday walk in the woods as a move toward their family, nature, health, and recreation. In other cases, they may notice choosing one of two or more potential toward moves. For example, on a Friday night they may notice choosing to stay home and declining an invitation to go out with friends as a move toward rest and self-care. Or faced with the same choice, they may notice choosing to go out with friends as a move toward friendship and recreation. (Also consider how these examples highlight the importance of function over form; after all, someone may notice staying home as a move away from tiredness, or going out with friends as a move away from guilt or being deemed a stick in the mud.)

After some time and multiple choices, people can look back upon their choices and notice whether the person they want to be would have chosen a similar balance of behaviors. If they notice that the person they want to be would have a different balance of choices, they can then notice how they choose in the coming days, weeks, and months.

Some folks may insist that values can be incompatible; for example, such as kindness and honesty. We've noticed that this mainly comes up in discussions between therapists. In our practice, we've found that it's best not to engage clients in these kinds of discussions about the content of values. Rather, we simply invite them to notice whether the person they want to be would want to embody one value without the other, or whether they'd ideally choose to somehow blend or combine them, alternate between them, or temper one with the other. There are a wealth of potential choices to notice, and it isn't particularly helpful to get verbally entangled with the apparent conflict.

In our clinical experience, clients typically don't stay stuck in so-called values conflicts for long, especially when we invite them to point at who or what is important, rather than describing their values with a lot of words.

In the Frame

As we have mentioned several times, deictic framing (I-you, here-there, now-then) is essential to perspective taking, so in this section we'll turn to how deictic framing is involved in the perspective-taking interview.

Perspective Taking as Central to Psychological Flexibility and Valued Living

At this point in the book, you're undoubtedly well aware that perspective taking is at the heart of matrix work. Simply stated, the matrix is a way to help people step back from their experience and see the big picture. As they sort with the matrix, they move to a perspective other than that from which they are experiencing things. As discussed in earlier chapters, this is basically deictic framing, which involves the ability to frame and discriminate three key perspectives: I-here-now versus you-there-then. Notice that these perspectives are all discriminations; that is, they involve noticing differences.

Recognizing these three discriminations is central to our ability to talk, understand, and be understood. Verbs in particular only become completely intelligible when conjugated to specify these perspectives. If you want to refer to an action with words, you can only do so intelligibly if you specify how the action is situated in time and space, and if you indicate who is or isn't performing the action.

The Value of Training a Reversal of Perspective

The deictic frames of I-you, here-there, and now-then have a number of important features that make them central to effective interventions and clinical practice. For example, when training psychological flexibility, it can be interesting to reverse these perspectives and invite clients to consider what they would experience if situated in a different place or time, or if they were someone else. So if you were standing where your partner is standing when the two of you argue, what would you see? Or, if you're stressed today and yesterday you were relaxed, what would you be experiencing if today was yesterday and yesterday was today? Or, if your partner wants you to share your difficulties and you feel that you should hide them, what would you want if your partner was you and you were your partner? Each of these questions prompts deictic framing.

Multiple exemplar training in perspective reversals using these kinds of questions has been shown to help children with developmental difficulties pass so-called theory of mind tests, which evaluate whether children are able to conceive of another person's perspective (McHugh & Stewart, 2012). In other words, these questions help people see the world through someone else's eyes.

The ability to take another person's perspective could be key to the ability to empathize with others (McHugh & Stewart, 2012). When you can experience things from another person's perspective, you gain access to his matrix, so to speak, allowing you to better notice both what is important to him and what painful inner stuff might get in the way. This makes it easier for you to connect with what he must be feeling, allowing you to feel sad when you notice that he's stuck and happy or excited if you notice that he's moving toward who or what is important to him.

Deictic Framing and the Matrix

Using the matrix activates perspective taking and deictic framing from the get-go, which, of course, sets the stage for the perspective-taking interview. People can only engage in sorting when they take a perspective that's somewhat distanced from what they're sorting. When people sort their experience on the matrix, they're doing so from the perspective of I-here-now looking at the experience of you-there-then, as mapped out on the matrix. In addition to helping people gain some distance from their experience, including sticky and painful stuff, it allows them to gain a more empathetic perspective on their own struggles. From this perspective, it's easier for them to self-validate and gently encourage themselves to engage in difficult toward moves. In this way, self-validation and self-compassion can emerge from deictic framing.

You could arguably think of the matrix and matrix work as based on training deictic framing and perspective taking. The matrix thus serves as a visual cue which, through deictic framing, can activate an entire network of relations that can change the functions of people's inner experience, helping shift them from getting stuck into away moves to being increasingly able to choose toward moves and build a valued life.

Deictic Framing from a First-Name Perspective

Though we currently don't have data on this, it seems plausible that verbal deictic framing could be a behavior engaged in from the perspective of one's first name. As a baby and toddler, you were repeatedly exposed to humans who used your first name to refer to you, as a mother does when she speaks to her child, perhaps saying, "Zaria is hungry" or "Zaria is eating an apple." Using the baby's given name in the third person makes sense, given that "me" and "you" are more complex because whom they refer to changes depending on the context and who is speaking and listening. Starting with first names (or a discrete term such as "Mom") establishes a basis for perspective taking using pointing. So a mother may repeatedly point at her baby saying "Zaria" and at herself saying "Mom." Only later will the mother and other caregivers train the relative perspectives of "me" and "you." Ultimately, emergence of the infant's given name as a referent is probably contemporaneous with developing ability to discriminate between the here-there spatial perspectives, the there-then temporal perspectives, and eventually the I-you perspectives.

This early learning history may facilitate later using one's first name to gain a third-person perspective on one's own experience. Absent clear data on this, our clinical explorations, initiated by Mark Webster, offer an intriguing vista into the potential inherent in inviting clients to use their first names when asking them to sort especially difficult stuff on the left side of their matrix. In other words, it may be most effective to guide a client to say, "Zaria's hook is fear. It comes with tightness in Zaria's chest, and when Zaria bites the hook, Zaria stops asking for what she wants."

This approach can also be useful when working with content on the right side of the matrix that feels inflexible. For example, say Zaria is hooked by the idea that she should take other people's needs into account (something she identifies as important and sorts on the right-hand side) and that when she bites that hook she doesn't ask for what she wants, which she sees as an away move because it meshes with a hook about feeling unimportant. In that case, you could invite her to use her first name in describing the dynamic: "Zaria can get hooked by how important it is to her to take other people's needs into account, and when Zaria bites that hook, Zaria doesn't ask for what she wants."

To speculate a bit more, it could be that moving from first name to first and last name may further increase perspective-taking. So for the preceding client, we might invite her to rephrase her first-name descriptions, this time using "Zaria Jones" to refer to herself. We believe this may be an effective way of training perspective taking. Try it and see how it works for you and your clients.

Ending Treatment

Once you've worked through the six steps with clients, they're likely to have developed enough psychological flexibility to end treatment. To assess this, consider using the psychological flexibility question (as also suggested at the end of chapter 4). You can simply ask, "Do you feel that you are now better able to choose to do what's important to you even in the presence of inner obstacles?" If the answer is yes, suggest that your work together might be coming to an end and offer to meet again in a month or two to check in on how things are going. If you want a more precise answer, invite clients to use a scale of 0 to 10 to evaluate the extent to which they feel they can engage in toward moves even in the presence of whatever shows up and gets in the way. You can ask them to provide a rating for both before therapy and at present, perhaps using the life dashboard worksheet, presented later in this book. In wrapping up, you might want to incorporate some of the other suggestions at the end of chapter 4, emphasizing that therapy isn't about never getting stuck again, but about getting unstuck faster. Also share some of the things you appreciate about your client and your work together.

Alternatively, if it seems that certain clients still need your support, by the end of the sixth step and the perspective-taking interview you'll have a good sense of which skills to target to enhance their flexibility and help them identify and engage in more workable behaviors. At this stage, you can go back and deliberately practice any of the steps. If you do need to practice some of the six steps in more depth, you may wish to bring a stronger focus on the therapeutic relationship by using the strategies outlined in chapter 7, if you haven't done so already.

Step 6 Checklist

Use this checklist (available for download at http://www.newharbinger.com /33605) to guide your practice of the strategies outlined in this chapter.

What I did

☐ I asked my client about how he had received the kittens of his distress since our previous session.

☐ I initiated the perspective-taking interview by inviting my client to choose a stuck situation that's likely to come.

☐ I first asked five-senses questions to make sure my client had identified a precise context, in time and space.

☐ I asked my client if he was there, in that future situation, before I invited him to imagine being teleported into the situation.

☐ I instructed my client to speak to his there-then perspective in the present tense.

☐ I asked my here-now client to see whether he could say something helpful to his there-then perspective.

☐ I used "you" to refer to my client's here-now perspective and his first name to refer to his there-then perspective.

☐ I made sure to ask my client how his there-then perspective received what the here-now client said to him.

☐ I guided my client in shifting perspectives a number of times.

☐ When I offered suggestions, they were very simple validating words offered to my here-now client to say to his there-then perspective.

☐ I asked my here-now client what his there-then perspective did next only after I noticed increased flexibility in the exchange.

☐ I invited my here-now client to estimate the probability that he would conduct a similar dialogue with his there-then self the next time the situation arises in real time.

☐ I invited my client to send me an e-mail or text message or otherwise let me know what he noticed when that stuck situation arises in real life.

What I didn't overdo

- ☐ Letting my client speak in the conditional
- ☐ Intervening in the conversation with my own suggestions beyond simply stated validations offered to my here-now client
- ☐ Suggesting convoluted forms of validation
- ☐ Engaging in any form of direct dialogue with the there-then perspective
- ☐ Insisting on a particular outcome

Concluding Words on the Six Steps

At heart, the matrix is neither a model nor a tool, much less a conceptual representation of human behavior or functioning. We feel it is best thought of as a visual cue that activates a functional contextual perspective on human experiences and behaviors. By inviting people to practice various discriminations, the matrix activates perspective taking and helps people contact broader aspects of both their five-senses and inner (predominantly verbal) experience, increasing the probability that they will engage in effective, workable behavior that moves them toward their values. In other words, the matrix cues psychological flexibility.

Another thing the matrix cues is noticing function rather than content or concepts. We have found this particularly valuable when training therapists. Using the matrix, therapists can hold concepts such as acceptance, defusion, and values more lightly and almost instantly notice function, rather than getting lost in trying to identify the "right" process or intervention.

The human mind naturally pulls all of us toward mechanistic rules—the world of right and wrong. The matrix, on the other hand, cues functional analysis and a pragmatic view of both context and behavior. Rather than providing or promoting rigid rules, the matrix points to context and workability, increasing our sensitivity to both and thereby enhancing our ability to flexibly track the broader consequences of our behaviors.

Because our minds pull us toward mechanistic rules, it should come as no surprise that developing a functional point of view can be extremely difficult to do. After all, from a functional contextual point of view, nothing *is* anything; things simply function as one thing or another depending on the context, and functions and contexts both continually change as they interact with one another. And for humans, the realm of verbal contexts exponentially multiplies the malleability of function and context. No wonder our minds tend to seek refuge in the apparent certainty of rules.

As matrix trainers, we've found that the hardest thing to convey to our trainees is how deep the functional contextual rabbit hole goes. There is literally no place to rest, and minds hate that. Yet as soon as we lose sight of the functional contextual viewpoint, we run the risk of looking for the "right" answer. In clinical work, this can take myriad forms, many of which involve trying to get clients to do things or see things a certain way. So as we arrive at the end of part 1 of the book, setting forth the six key steps for enhancing client flexibility, let's take a look at a few aspects of the matrix that can help you, the clinician, enhance your own flexibility as a matrix practitioner.

The Matrix Isn't About Getting Anyone to Do Anything

The matrix isn't about getting clients to do anything, nor is it about getting you to do anything. It's about getting you and your clients to explore a point of view and notice what shows up. Use it to point to clients' experience. Because you don't have direct access to their experience, your task is more about noticing the signs that clients are noticing their experience than about getting them to notice anything in particular. In other words, this work is more about the function of your pointing than the form of your pointing or the form of what clients experience when you point.

Of course, the matrix isn't a miracle cure for the human condition. When using it, you'll still get hooked. We know we do, even on our good days. And when you get hooked, you may start using the matrix in a mechanistic way, trying to get clients to see, say, or do something you believe they should see, say, or do. That isn't a problem as long as you notice it and get unhooked—or at least notice that you're hooked and what you do next.

A Shortcut for Keeping It Functional

One of the most effective ways to get unhooked is to share your matrix with clients. And because we all get hooked, we hope that after reading this you'll notice yourself sharing your matrix with your clients on a regular basis. If you don't, it may be that you don't notice getting hooked. And whether or not you get hooked, sharing your matrix can be an effective way to keep the focus on function, as it involves sharing what shows up for you in the moment: the present functions of the present-moment context—including the client's behavior—as it interacts with your history and verbal context. This will give you some perspective on your own experience, enhancing your flexibility and allowing you to model these processes for clients.

An effective follow-up is to ask clients to respond by showing you what they notice showing up in their matrix when you share yours. We'll delve into this in chapter 7, as we explore how you can use the therapeutic relationship to enhance clients' ability to create and nurture deep and satisfying relationships.

Creating Tailor-Made Discriminations

The six steps in part 1 of this book train clients in various basic discriminations. We present them in a sequence in which they build on one another in a way that we have found useful in training and in our clinical practice. This doesn't mean that you must use these and only these discriminations or that you must use them in this precise order for all of your clients, regardless of their presentation and context.

Once you understand that discrimination training is at the heart of the six steps, you may start noticing which discriminations will work best for a particular client. As you may have guessed, we believe that a key discrimination is between behavior to move toward who or what is important and behavior to move away or under the control of what we get hooked by. We are currently in the process of empirically testing this hypothesis.

That said, no discrimination is in itself sacred. The right discrimination is the one that works in the context in which it is used. So in training self-compassion, you might use moving toward and moving away in the abstract, as ways of approaching one's aversive inner experience and self-judgments, even though these behaviors are largely internal and not observable. What makes it appropriate to use the terms "toward move" and "away move" in this context is that those terms can help transform the aversive functions of these experiences and judgments on a client's observable behaviors, as well as on the client's sense of well-being.

So as you become familiar with the six-step approach in this book, be creative and be sure to take your cues from clients' language to come up with discriminations that work. It isn't even necessary to use the "toward" versus "away" discrimination. It could be equally or more effective to use a discrimination between moving toward being right and moving toward who or what is important. Always remember that none of the terms we suggest are used in a conceptual sense; they are used in a functional way and stand or fall depending on the function they have in the context in which they are used.

To be clear, sticking to the discriminations outlined in the six steps when they aren't working is a sign of a mechanistic use of the matrix, and thus a sign that even though the approach outwardly resembles matrix work, it no longer has that function. If it seems that we're belaboring this point, it's a risk we're willing to take, as our experience has been that this is the point most people, including experienced ACT therapists, can misunderstand about using the matrix.

The Matrix Without the Matrix

The matrix isn't a thing, and matrix work isn't about the matrix. At heart, it's about taking a functional contextual perspective on one's behavior and experience. To prompt that perspective-taking behavior, think of the matrix as a cue that can be gradually phased out. As a matter of fact, you may have noticed that steps 5 and 6 can be practiced without explicit reference to the matrix. This is deliberate and helps ensure that clients can learn to notice the difference between moving toward and moving away absent a matrix. Thinking of the matrix as a cue can also help you consider cueing again when clients—or you—experience particular difficulties in using the functional contextual point of view.

Advanced matrix work can thus completely eschew the matrix, looking for all the world like nonmatrix work. For example, you could practice this work through extensive yessing and systematically redirecting clients' attention to what they do, feel, and think, to who or what is important, and to what they do when all of this shows up. You may never show them the matrix or mention it, and yet you'd still be doing matrix work, as matrix work is not the matrix. We'll leave this at that koan.

PART 2

The Matrix and the Social World

In part 1 of the book, we outlined how to use the matrix to help individuals get unstuck, including learning how to get unstuck on their own. In part 2, we turn to the wider social world. Chapter 7 delves into using the matrix in therapeutic relationship–focused work. Chapters 8 through 10 are devoted to using the matrix when working with parents and children, with couples, and in life coaching, respectively; you might think of these as prosocial uses of the matrix. Then, in the final chapter, we offer guidance on how to incorporate the matrix into other approaches, from CBT and schema therapy to motivational interviewing and psychodynamic therapy.

CHAPTER 7

Using the Therapeutic Relationship in Matrix Work

The matrix is a tool to help people get unstuck. In our experience, the six steps outlined in part 1, whether you deliver them as six sequential sessions or in some other way, usually do a fairly comprehensive job of retraining clients' relationship with their inner experience in such a way that they are better able to choose to do what's important to them even in the presence of inner obstacles. In other words, those six steps are quite effective in training psychological flexibility.

It may seem as though matrix work is largely intrapersonal, with a focus on processes that are internal to individuals trained with the matrix. However, as we'll explore in part 2 of the book, the matrix is also a powerful tool for promoting flexibility and values-congruent behavior in relationships. In subsequent chapters, we'll delve into using the matrix with families and couples. In this chapter, we'll establish what can serve as a foundation for that work: using the matrix, the six steps, and the therapeutic relationship to help clients develop interpersonal skills and work toward their relationship goals and values. This approach integrates many strategies from functional analytic psychotherapy (FAP; Kohlenberg & Tsai, 1991), a close cousin of ACT that focuses on the therapeutic relationship and training interpersonal behavior in the moment, in session, to help clients move toward the life and relationships they want.

Social Stuck Loops

When we're stuck in away moves, it's difficult to connect deeply with others. Our lives are dominated by attempts to avoid discomfort or pain or consumed by other behaviors that can interfere with relationships, such as seeking to be right, self-isolation, or being overly passive. Authentic interactions with others take second place. Yet humans are a highly social species, and relationships with others are often at the top of people's list of what's important. This is why we choose to ask "Who is important?" before "What is important?"; for most people, relationships are what comes first. Therefore, one of the many advantages of liberating ourselves from stuck loops is that it allows us to turn toward building more satisfying relationships.

For many clients, the six steps in part 1 are sufficient to facilitate turning toward those who are important; in other words, they facilitate relationship-oriented toward moves. If these clients are well integrated into a relatively healthy social environment, their toward moves will naturally be reinforced by others, and your work together may come to an end with no need to focus more directly on interpersonal relating.

Unfortunately, real life often isn't that neat. Everyone has their own hooks, habitual away moves, and stuck loops, and the interactions between one person's hooked behavior and another's can keep not just individuals but also their relationships stuck. When one person engages in an away move in the context of a relationship, that away move may become a hook for the other person, who is likely to respond with an away move too. For example, a woman may be easily hooked by the thought that her needs don't deserve consideration. So when her husband asks where she'd like to go out to eat, she may bite that hook and, instead of expressing what she wants, say, "Wherever you like," in a passive, resigned way. This response may hook her husband, who bites by choosing to go out with friends instead, leaving her at home. This could feed her idea that her needs don't deserve consideration, fueling a vicious cycle. This kind of dynamic can keep relationships firmly on the left side of the matrix, draining them of vitality and increasing the likelihood of fruitless conflict.

Another issue is that some people are so deeply stuck that they have become desocialized and isolated or are caught in a web of dysfunctional relationships. In the latter case, whatever toward moves they're able to make in their relationships may go unnoticed or, worse, be punished by others.

Finally, and sadly, some children are raised in environments dominated by stuck relationship loops and lack experience with relationships in which toward moves are encouraged and reinforced, so even as adults they may lack crucial interpersonal skills. These are people who will especially benefit from a deliberate focus on interpersonal relationships, in addition to the six basic matrix steps.

The Importance of Cooperating and Relating

To set a context for why therapeutic relationship–focused work can be so effective, let's take a quick look at the history and current context of human social relating and how language is involved in that. Humans are the most social of all primates. This is another result of the double-edged sword of language. In addition to helping us control the outer world, language is responsible for our amazing ability to cooperate with one another. Without it, we wouldn't have been able to cooperate to develop and refine our technologies as we have, nor would we be able to share in such an exquisitely detailed way the ever-changing nuances of our inner experience. Cooperation is as essential to human well-being as it is to human survival. And language is our prime tool of cooperation.

Complex human societies evolved from bands and tribes. Although tribes are largely cooperative internally, they often compete—at times to the death—with other bands of humans for access to scarce resources. When tribal bonds were strong, it was easy to discriminate between people who were a likely source of comfort and safety (tribe members) and those who represented a potential threat (all others). Furthermore, because inclusion in the tribe was a condition of survival for individual members, our ancestors naturally grew extremely sensitive to the threat of rejection from the group—a sensitivity to social exclusion we retain to this day. However, most of us no longer have strong group bonds akin to those that exist in tribes, and we are also potentially able to be in contact with vast numbers of other humans. Therefore, every individual can represent either a source of great comfort and safety or a looming threat of social exclusion (or worse).

In such a context, opportunities to establish profound intimate bonds in which to share our deepest thoughts and feelings without fear of rejection become highly appetitive. If you know what the people closest to you really think and feel, you are better able to predict their behavior, and that in itself may be a highly prized source of comfort and safety. That sense of safety is probably one of the conditions that allows humans to bond deeply with one another. When, on the other hand, people don't know how to recognize, create, and nurture such relationships, they are more vulnerable to the entire range of mental and personality disorders. The therapeutic relationship can offer an ideal context for the needed learning when it has been absent from a client's personal history.

Returning to language, let's examine the role of transformation of functions (which is part and parcel of language) in the arc of human social development outlined just above. The process of transformation of functions, in which mental experience can carry some of the functions of five-senses experience, allowed humans to build abstract models of the world and test them by experience, helping us develop increasingly sophisticated means of cooperating and of controlling the outer world. Yet it also gave rise to a mental world in which we can be trapped by imagined threats or foibles, such as a strong need to be right, and lose sight of the impact of our behavior on others. For many people, this has led to retreating to a world of inner and mental experience, disconnected from others yet pervaded by a longing for deep and stable connection, as indicated by the centrality of love and family bonds in most human cultures. That social connection is so central seems to be confirmed by a recent meta-analysis that identified social isolation as a major risk factor for early death, on a par with smoking and higher than drinking (Holt-Lunstad, Smith, & Layton, 2010). Apparently, the ability to create and maintain intimate relationships is central not only to mental health, but to general well-being. In this light, it isn't surprising that, clinically, the question "Who is important?" almost always elicits answers.

Defining Intimacy

We would define an intimate relationship along the lines of Cordova and Scott (2001): as one in which you are mostly reinforced and rarely punished for sharing what you think and feel and in turn mostly reinforce and rarely punish the other person for doing the same. This definition distinguishes intimate relationships from romantic relationships, which are based on mutual sexual attraction and preoccupation with the object of one's affection. Intimate relating is based on authenticity, caring for the other person, and validating the person's experience, and the ability to relate in this way probably underlies satisfying friendships and family relationships. Thus, it is a crucial skill for forming the deep bonds that are such an important component of well-being.

Creating a Context for Learning Intimate Relating

Therapy naturally gravitates around clients' personal experience. In ACT, we seek to help clients receive whatever they think and feel without getting hooked by it. When you practice yessing, this helps create the conditions of an intimate relationship. It's a way of ensuring that you mostly reinforce and rarely punish clients for sharing what they think and feel—the first element of relating intimately. To get to full intimate relating with a given client, that client would also have to mostly reinforce and rarely punish you for sharing what you think and feel. Learning this skill is immensely helpful to clients in forging and nurturing the relationships they long for.

Within ACT, the therapeutic relationship (and, more broadly, the therapeutic context) is ideally suited for this kind of work. Such work is best primed by creating an explicitly intimate context. You can do this by telling clients that, in the service of helping them create and nurture the kinds of relationships they want, you're committed to making space for everything they think and feel and to being authentic whenever you share what you think and feel. In chapter 1, in the section on informed consent, we outlined a metaphor of waves that's helpful for letting clients know that the difficulties they experience in day-to-day life may show up in your sessions or even in your relationship. As recommended in chapter 1, let clients know that this is not only normal and acceptable, but can also provide precious opportunities for them to notice their experience and authentically share what they think and feel. Also explain that this will give them a chance to practice building the kinds of relationships they want.

Once you obtain client consent for this kind of therapeutic relationship–focused work, get permission to ask whether something the client is doing, feeling, or thinking in interactions with you may also show up at other times and with other people. Also make it clear that the client is the only expert on her experience, so you will always defer to her perspective and let go of any of your own thoughts that prove unhelpful.

As you engage in therapeutic relationship–focused work, stay attentive to the experience and processes of intimate relating and hone your awareness of opportunities to encourage clients to practice intimate relating. Also understand that doing this work means having the courage to engage in intimate relating with clients and caring and loving them enough to create a deeply authentic and supportive relationship with them. This directly reflects the stance in functional analytic psychotherapy, wherein awareness, courage, and love are central processes in both intimate relating and therapeutic change (Tsai et al., 2009).

Using an Interpersonal Focus to Help Clients Get Unstuck

Beyond helping clients develop the kinds of relationships they want, there are other reasons why you may want to remain aware of interpersonal processes that arise in session and use the therapeutic relationship itself as a tool for clinical change. Key among them is that using the six steps without noticing and attending to what's going on in the therapeutic relationship and how it relates to clients' difficulties in everyday life may hinder progress.

Other reasons relate to creating an optimal learning environment. As mentioned, learning new behavior can only be done in the present moment, and it requires practice. Pretty much the only thing we can do outside of the present moment in relation to learning is to talk about past or future practice—and there's a huge difference between talking about doing something and actually doing it. This is the problem with therapy that focuses exclusively on clients' lives outside of sessions; it's likely to be an exercise in talking about stuff, rather than training new behavior that could help clients get unstuck.

Another reason to focus on the therapeutic relationship has to do with how people respond to learning environments. People generally seek therapy in an effort to learn how to better handle things. Therapy is thus a learning environment. In a learning environment, people are presented with instructions and invited to practice new behavior. However, not everyone who enters therapy is apt to take instructions and try out new behaviors. In chapter 5, we described the impacts of early rule-giving contexts on people. One impact of certain contexts is to make most learning environments—and verbal rules in particular—aversive. So some clients' difficulties may be rooted in the way they react to instructions. This is something you can work on in the moment in the context of the therapeutic relationship.

Finally, some clients who come into therapy are so stuck in their lives that at first it may be exceedingly difficult for them to try new behaviors, especially if they're asked to do so outside of session. Such clients are best served by focusing on whatever is present in the moment, including the therapeutic relationship and the impact the therapist and client have on one another.

In this work, and in therapy in general, keep an eye out for when something happens between you and the client that suddenly makes you lose her. You may see her visibly shut down or strongly react to something you said or did, or you may not see much but feel that things have screeched to a halt. For some reason, the client has stopped engaging in learning. Maybe you did or said something that made her bite a familiar hook. Maybe she experiences so many hooks around learning that your work together causes her to shut down, making it hard for any learning to take place. In such cases, it's especially appropriate and effective to look at what's going on in the present moment. Often that means looking at what's going on in the therapeutic relationship.

Clinically Relevant Behavior

Functional analytic psychotherapy is based on the same functional contextual point of view as ACT. FAP focuses largely on the therapeutic relationship and the interpersonal behaviors that occur in sessions. Of particular interest are *clinically relevant behaviors* (CRBs)—behaviors that occur in session and in the context of the therapeutic relationship that are clinically relevant in the sense that they are exemplars, on one hand, of the client's real-life problematic behavior (termed CRB1) and, on the other hand, of the client's real-life improved behavior (termed CRB2). Translated into matrix terms, CRBs are the away moves and toward moves clients engage in during sessions (Schoendorff & Bolduc, 2014).

A Functional Definition of Clinically Relevant Behavior

Central to the definition of CRBs is that these behaviors take place in session. Further, they aren't defined by their outward appearance. What makes them clinically relevant is that they share the same functions as the targeted real-life behavior. Here's an example: If a client describes how she avoided asking her boss for a raise, avoiding asking her boss for a raise isn't clinically relevant behavior, as it didn't take place in session. On the other hand, if the client is avoiding talking to you about her financial difficulties and how they might impact her ability to pay for therapy, this would be clinically relevant behavior because it's an exemplar of the same behavior as not asking her boss for a raise.

Further, it is not so much the subject of the discussion (money) that makes the client's in-session avoidance an instance of CRB; rather, it is her difficulty in asking for her needs to be met. Ultimately, the function or consequence of this behavior is that the client's needs are indeed unlikely to be met, due to her behaviors. So for a behavior to be clinically relevant, it has to occur both in session and in the client's life outside of session. Further, a behavior is clinically relevant not because its form is necessarily the same when it occurs in session and outside, but because its functions are the same in and out of session.

This focus on function rather than form invites therapists to consider broader classes of behavior, beyond individual actions. For interpersonal behaviors, proponents of FAP have proposed five classes that can lead to clinically relevant behavior (Callaghan, 2001):

- Assertion of needs

- Bidirectional communication

- Conflict

- Disclosure and interpersonal closeness

- Emotional experience and expression

Glenn Callaghan (2006) offers a 117-item questionnaire (now reduced to 111 items; Darrow, Callaghan, Bonow, & Follette, 2014) to assist therapists in assessing clients' interpersonal behaviors and skills. We feel that giving clients a 111-item questionnaire may be a bit unwieldy; however, it can be useful to keep these five broad classes of behavior in mind as you work with clients. This will help you more readily notice CRBs when they occur so that you can work with them. It will also help you remember that CRBs are defined by their function, not their form.

Viewing Clinically Relevant Behavior Through the Matrix

From a matrix perspective, clinically relevant behaviors are sorted as toward and away moves that occur in session. For clients, looking at their experience through the entire matrix, as when practicing verbal aikido, readily becomes a toward move that's likely to help them get unstuck. And if they practice noticing with the matrix point of view when facing difficulties in everyday life, they're more likely to choose toward moves. In other words, looking through the matrix is CRB2. Conversely, not looking at their experience through the matrix could be seen as CRB1, or an away move, and this behavior is likely to keep them stuck in everyday life.

Your mind may be quick to notice CRB1. When this happens, it's perfectly okay to ask clients for permission to share the thoughts that showed up for you. However, if a client doesn't concur with your suggestion, it's best to drop it, as it doesn't reflect the client's experience. And even if your insight is on track, if the client doesn't concur, it's unlikely that the two of you can effectively work on that behavior in the moment. So be prepared to drop any interpretation that clients don't validate. Don't worry too much about missing the real problem; after all, if it's a real problem, it won't miss you.

One way to assure more neutrality on your part is to notice potential CRBs (both CRB1 and CRB2) in session and then ask whether the client sees a given behavior as more of a toward or an away move. Be sure to ask this question in regard to both classes of CRB. If you only ask it when you think clients are engaged in away moves, the question itself may become aversive. Then, instead of prompting noticing, it may prompt more away moves. So be sure to take a balanced approach and also ask this question when clients appear to be engaging in toward moves.

More broadly, matrix work tends to support CRB2, as looking through the matrix invites clients to look at the whole of their context and behavioral choices. When this is generalized to everyday life, it will increase valued living. The neat thing about this is that looking through the matrix is a behavior that can be trained in session, regardless of what you and the client are looking at, whether past situations, imagined future situations, or what's going on in the present moment and the therapeutic relationship. Further, using the matrix in session can increase the probability that the client will generalize the newly trained behavior, because all that's required is exporting the same behavior: looking through the matrix, regardless of context.

Working with clinically relevant behavior in session can supercharge your therapeutic work, increasing focus and intensity. It also multiplies clients' opportunities to learn more adaptive interpersonal behaviors and gives them a chance to practice toward moves when they would otherwise automatically engage in away moves. If you're like us, seeing clients engage in toward moves in situations where they formerly would have engaged in away moves will make your heart sing. If this happens, share that with your client. Doing so will naturally reinforce toward moves.

Identifying CRB1 and CRB2 in the Present Moment

As we've said many times, in matrix work, the key is to get clients to notice their away moves (CRB1) and toward moves (CRB2), as well as the inner experiences that can drive them. To identify these moves when they occur in session so that they can serve as present-moment instances of the behavior to work on in the moment, pay as close attention to what clients are doing as to what they are talking about. For example, a client may have shared her feeling that nobody understands her. Then, you may subsequently notice her talking at a rushed pace and in such a roundabout way that it's difficult for you to follow her. Keeping in mind the essential matrix practice of pointing to the clients' own experience, you might gently ask her if the way she talks about her difficulty is more of a toward move or an away move. You could also share your experience of finding it difficult to follow her and ask whether she thinks other people may have a similar experience. In other words, you would share some of what shows up in your matrix while inviting your client to validate a possible parallel between what's happening between you in session and what may occur in her life outside. This is a key move for jointly identifying CRB.

Sharing your own matrix may make it easier for the client to notice the effect her behavior has on you and, presumably, on others around her. We are very deliberate in saying "presumably." After all, there's always the possibility that the effect this client has on you is more an effect of your own history than a function of her behavior. If you think this could be the case, it's probably best to ask the client. For example, we know of a therapist who had a history of feeling bored whenever he spoke with his sister. As it happened, he found himself working with a client who looked a lot like his sister and even spoke like her. So when he started feeling bored, he thought that must be due to his own history and how he related to his sister. They proceeded through the six steps and the client made good progress in terms of increasing her toward moves. However, she was still unhappy in her interpersonal relationships, both with her husband and with her colleagues. Then one day the therapist summoned up the courage to reveal his own matrix—specifically his inner experience of having trouble following the client. The following dialogue reveals how fruitful this was.

Therapist: (*Interrupts a long, rambling monologue.*) May I take a risk right now?

Client: Sure.

Therapist: How can I say this? At times, when you speak I feel as though we're adrift at sea. Every now and again it feels like you grab on to a rock for a few seconds, but then you let go of it and we drift some more, until you grab the next rock. It's a toward move for me to let you know this. Do you think others may feel something similar when you speak with them?

Client: Well, I do notice a lot of blank stares.

Therapist: Would you like to find a way to interact with people that doesn't make them feel what I described?

Client: Sure.

Therapist: Okay, so let's see if we can find a name for this way of speaking.

Client: I don't know. Being boring?

Therapist: That feels too harsh. Any other ideas?

Client: What about…sliding?

Therapist: Sliding could work. It's neutral enough. Would you sort sliding as more of a toward move or an away?

Client: Definitely away. Part of it is that I'm afraid I don't cover all of the bases, and part of it is that I feel I have to explain everything or I'll be misunderstood. So it's a move away from that.

Therapist: Great. And are you noticing that we've been sliding much since we started talking about sliding?

Client: Not much.

Therapist: Me neither. How about we keep an eye on the sliding in our exchanges today?

Client: Okay, let's do that.

In the rest of this session, there was much less "sliding." From then on, both therapist and client kept an eye out for this way of speaking, which began to diminish both in session and in the client's life. After two more sessions, the client reported that she was connecting more deeply with her husband and colleagues. She also reported having been able to turn down offers of extra work, which in the past she'd always found herself accepting after much "sliding." The moral of this story is that the best way to know whether clients' impact on you is representative of how they impact others is to simply ask, pretty much regardless of what your mind tells you regarding the origins of what you feel.

To use this approach in your own practice, think of an amplifier with two volume knobs, one for the lower left of your matrix and one for the lower right. Whenever clients do something that activates the lower right quadrant of your matrix, don't hesitate to turn the volume up. The worst that can happen is that a client has trouble receiving your positive regard (possibly a CRB1), which may be something to work on. When clients activate the lower left quadrant of your matrix, first choose whether to share this. Because this can be delicate and is likely to be aversive for clients, don't rush into it, and always ask for permission first. Also, be careful not to say that anything that may work to your client's detriment and weaken intimacy between the two of you. Then, if you do choose to share some of what's going on in the lower left quadrant of your matrix, turn the volume down low. The worst that can happen is that the client doesn't hear you, in which case you can increase the volume. However, if the signal is too loud at first, this may have aversive functions for the client, which could have highly unfortunate consequences. If hearing you has been too aversive, she may move away from therapy altogether.

Using Awareness, Courage, and Love with the Matrix

Functional analytic psychotherapy is sometimes presented as comprising three central processes: awareness, courage, and love. In FAP, awareness, courage, and love are both the processes the therapist uses and the skills in which clients are trained. In this context, awareness means noticing CRBs and our impacts on others. Courage is about engaging in behavior in line with our values, speaking our truth, and sharing our thoughts and feelings, including about how other people's behavior affects us. And love refers to speaking and acting with kindness and compassion and supporting and reinforcing bids for connection.

By now, it should be abundantly clear that the matrix is a tool for promoting awareness, which can help people get unstuck in relation to their values and life goals. Courage and love are, of course, central ingredients in helping people improve their interpersonal relationships. Many clients find it difficult to muster the courage to speak their truth, or if they do, they fail to speak in a way that's loving enough that others are able to hear, receive, and act on what they've shared. When engaging in therapeutic relationship–focused work, it can be useful to present these cornerstones of awareness, courage, and love to clients, describing courage and love as two classes of toward moves they could notice choosing in the service of improving their relationships.

The dialogue below provides an illustration of using this approach with Patty, a client meeting criteria for borderline personality disorder. She made good strides with the six basic matrix steps, and now she and her therapist are engaged in deeper therapeutic relationship–focused work.

Therapist: Since we've started our work together, you've become pretty skilled at looking at difficult situations through the matrix, and it's been a joy to see you get unstuck in so many situations. As we discussed in our previous session, now could be a good time to start working on your relationships. We can do this by paying attention to what goes on in the moment in our relationship here and by using the matrix to help you move toward your relationship goals. Moving toward satisfying and long-lasting relationships requires three key skills: awareness, courage, and love. Awareness is essentially looking through your matrix and noticing your impacts on others. Courage has to do with speaking your truth and taking a chance on interpersonal toward moves. And love has to do with meeting others with kindness and compassion and supporting them in their toward moves. Where would you put courage and love in your matrix?

Client: In the top right, I guess.

Therapist: Excellent. So let's do that and let's see if you can identify some courage and love toward moves you can engage in, either here with me, in your life out there, or both. We'll just list them, and then you can see if you notice choosing to engage in any of them either here, today, or between now and our next session.

Client: For courage, I could tell my mom that I need her to simply validate me when I feel bad and not try to solve my problems. I could say the same to my friend Tracy.

Therapist: Cool. And how about here with me?

Client: Well, I could tell you when I feel you're going too fast or not connecting with me.

Therapist: Great. Is it happening now?

Client: It was a minute ago, but it's better now.

Therapist: Wow, thanks for taking the risk of telling me. I'll try to go more slowly. (Pauses.) Any more courage moves?

Client: I could tell my boss that I'm struggling with the new project. And more generally, I could try to express my needs more.

Therapist: Great. That's a pretty good set of courage moves. Let's look at love now. What loving behaviors could you do here with me, out there between now and our next session, or both?

Client: (Blushes and chuckles.) I could tell you how much you've helped me already and show my appreciation.

Therapist: Oh, thanks. That's sweet. You've worked so hard, and I feel honored to do this work with you.

Client: I could let my mom know her support is important to me. I could be kinder to my son. Generally, I could share more appreciation with people; for example, at work.

Therapist: Okay, we've got a pretty good list already. I'll give you this list to take home with you so you can see what you notice around doing or not doing these toward moves—or other courage and love toward moves you may notice.

In the next session, Patty reported that she'd noticed engaging in quite a few courage and love toward moves. A number of them were similar to those she'd done in session, such as expressing her needs and sharing her appreciation of others. She was also eager to come up with more courage and love toward moves.

In our clinical practice, we've found that clients readily take to incorporating courage and love in this way, and that it can be an effective tool to draw their attention toward key interpersonal behaviors. As you proceed with this work, help clients calibrate new courage and love toward moves so they continue to step outside of their comfort zone while remaining inside their self-care zone. We've included an illustration (figure 8) that you can use when doing this work with clients (available for download at http://www.newharbinger.com/33605).

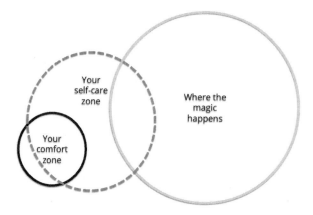

Figure 8.

Here's how you might present this approach.

Therapist: As you start trying more of these courage and love toward moves, it's important to step outside your comfort zone, but also to take care of yourself. To help you do this, let's look at the relationship between three important zones: your comfort zone, the zone where the magic happens, and your self-care zone. Within your comfort zone are the toward moves you're already doing without much effort. Those are great. However, you can't learn new toward moves or become more effective in moving toward what you care about if you stay in your comfort zone. The magic happens some distance outside of your comfort zone, and it isn't possible to know the precise distance between the two. So you simply have to start moving outside your comfort zone. As you do so, see if you can remain inside your self-care zone—the zone where you make sure you take workable risks and are kind to yourself. Your self-care zone is probably larger than your comfort zone, so try to notice that zone outside your comfort zone and inside your self-care zone where the magic happens, then aim for this sweet spot. Can you notice where that is for you?

After you've introduced this image, when clients identify toward moves, be sure to ask whether those moves are outside of their comfort zone and whether they're inside their self-care zone. If the answer to the first question is no, ask whether they'd be willing to take a bigger step outside their comfort zone. If the answer to the second question is no, ask whether they can take a smaller step so they remain inside their self-care zone. By calibrating potential toward moves with clients in this way, you let them know that they matter to you and that you're putting them at the center of the work. You also help them learn to assess risk and how much risk is workable given their current context and skills.

The Five Rules of FAP

We've almost completed our primer in the FAP principles that inform our matrix approach to therapeutic relationship–focused work. The final piece we'll share is what's known as the five rules of FAP (Tsai et al., 2009). These rules basically delineate a stepwise process for working with CRB using courage, awareness, and love, so you may find it useful to keep them in mind as you do this work with clients. For each, we'll address how that rule relates to processes inherent in matrix work.

Rule 1. Notice CRB. This is an awareness rule. By becoming aware of clients' CRBs, you can help them notice these behaviors. Matrix work takes a similar approach by asking clients (and clinicians) whether a given behavior is more of a toward or away move and whether that behavior also shows up outside of session.

Rule 2. Evoke CRB. This is a courage rule. You can help bring CRB into the room by inviting clients to engage in a behavior that's difficult for them. This seldom requires a stretch, as CRB can be evoked by the very nature of therapy: the fee structure, setting an agenda, recommending home practice exercises, ending therapy, and so on. From a matrix perspective, asking clients to sort into the matrix will bring CRB into the room by giving clients an opportunity to engage in either a CRB2 by sorting or a CRB1 by not sorting.

Rule 3. Respond contingently to CRB and naturally reinforce CRB2. This is a love rule, because reinforcing people when they move toward their goals (and being reinforced by the fact that they're doing this) is part of what love is. When clients produce CRB1, you can respond contingently by blocking it or by seeking to shape the part of their behavior that could become a toward move. However, blocking CRB1 can be aversive to clients, so make sure you ask for permission, and then be as gentle as you can and offer an alternative toward move your client could engage in. For example, with a client who talks incessantly, you could ask if the two of you might take a breath together and then reinforce your client for pausing. When clients produce CRB2, you can reinforce this by responding appropriately and letting them know how you feel when you see them make progress. For example, if a client expresses her need for you to adjust your fee, and for her expressing a need is CRB2, you could reinforce this by lowering your fee and by telling her how happy you are to see her ask for what she needs. From a matrix perspective, whenever you notice clients engaging in the CRB2 of noticing through their matrix, let them know you've noticed and appreciate this.

Rule 4. Notice the effects of your behavior on clients. This is an awareness rule, as it involves being aware of your impacts. Everyone responds differently, and what may be reinforcing for one client may be punishing for another. You'll know whether your behavior has been reinforcing if a client does more of the behavior you've tried to reinforce—not just in the short term, but also in the long term. Technically, you can only know if reinforcement is effective by observing whether the target behavior increases. However, it's also a good idea to ask clients how things went for them. Another way to work with this rule is to ask clients to share appreciations at the end of a session. Your appreciations can further reinforce CRB2, and the client's appreciations can give you insight into whether your behavior is achieving the desired effect. Plus, by asking clients how things went for them, you model being aware of one's impact, a skill that can only help your clients in their interpersonal interactions.

Rule 5. Provide functional explanations and promote generalization. This is an awareness and courage rule. The matrix is an ideal tool for practicing functional analysis: the identification of antecedents, behavior, and consequence (the ABC model). Its flexibility allows you to choose whether the relevant antecedent to a behavior is an event in the world of the five senses, as in traditional behavior analysis, or a private event, like a thought or emotion. Similarly, the behavior can be either an observable toward or away move or a covert behavior, such as ruminating. Finally, the consequence can be either the actual toward or away behavior or what happens in the world outside the skin after clients engage in either a toward or away move. In contrast with traditional ABC models, this way of conducting a functional analysis is nonlinear, making it easier to grasp that "antecedent," "behavior," and "consequences" are ways of looking at events, rather than things in themselves. This can help clients get how their behavior can become an antecedent for the behavior of others, particularly when it hooks others.

Verbal Aikido for Two

Engaging in verbal aikido for two is an excellent way to work with interpersonal functions in the room. This differs from verbal aikido as described in chapter 4 in that the therapist also answers the seven basic questions. You can use the Verbal Aikido for Two Worksheet for this if you like (available for download at http://www.newharbinger.com/33605).

We'll illustrate verbal aikido through a dialogue with Sam, a client who came in therapy to work on his anxiety. After going through the first five steps of matrix work, Sam shared that it all felt too theoretical and that he wanted to practice the matrix skills in real time. As you'll see, verbal aikido for two is great for this because it provides a context for the therapist to engage in the practice and model the skills. (Note that the proviso from chapter 4 applies to all forms of verbal aikido, including verbal aikido for two: the question numbers are included here solely for ease of presentation; in actual practice they aren't used, and it isn't necessary to go through them in sequence if the context calls for using them more flexibly.)

Therapist: I think it's a really good idea to practice in real time. Would you like to try verbal aikido for two? It's the same as the verbal aikido you've already practiced, except I'll practice along with you. We can use this Verbal Aikido for Two Worksheet as we go. On the worksheet, one matrix is yours and the other is mine. During our exchange, we'll each point to our basic moves on our respective matrices. Okay?

Client: Okay.

Therapist: So would you like me to start?

Client: You start.

Therapist: Okay. With my five senses (*pointing to question 1*), I heard your words about how this feels too theoretical and you want some real-time practice. I noticed some hooks (*pointing to question 2*) about not being good enough—thoughts like "This isn't working," "I'm not a good therapist for you," and "I hope he doesn't quit." I noticed some shame and (*pointing to question 3*) some queasiness and constriction in the back of my throat (*pointing to her throat*). If I had bitten those hooks, you would have seen me start the session with something else (*pointing to question 4*). I chose to actively work with it (*pointing to question 5*) because the therapist I want to be would respond to your request. What's important to me about that (*pointing to question 6*) is to serve you the best I can and to be open and responsive (*pointing to question 7*). It feels like a bit of a flutter in my upper chest (*pointing to her chest*). Okay, now it's your turn. See if you can respond to what I just said using the verbal aikido moves and pointing to your matrix and your body.

Client: Okay. So I'm happy that you're responding to my request.

Therapist: And where does that go?

Client: There (*pointing to question 6*).

Therapist: Cool. Do you notice any hooks?

Client: Yes, I notice feeling embarrassed and not being sure what to say. So those go here (*pointing to question 2*). And it feels a bit weird here (*pointing to his upper belly*). If I bit the hook (*pointing to question 4*), what would you see me do? Maybe just talk without using this (*tapping on the worksheet*). And what would the person I want to be do? I guess what you're seeing me doing right now (*pointing to question 5*). And what's important to me in doing that (*pointing to question 6*)? To really get this, I guess. As for how that feels and where I feel it in my body (*pointing to question 7*), it feels good. I'm not sure where that is in my body. Maybe here (*pointing to his chest*).

Therapist: Great! So for me the hook right now (*pointing to question 2*) is that this feels like such an unnatural way of speaking and I'm afraid you may find it useless. It's most intense here (*pointing to her upper belly*). If I bit the hook (*pointing to question 4*), you would see me drop this conversation. The therapist I want to be (*pointing to question 5*) sticks with it and asks you how exchanging in this way makes you feel. What's important to me in doing that (*pointing to question 6*) is to make sure you get really fluid at this practice. This feels warm in my chest (*pointing at question 7, then pointing at her chest*).

Before we continue this dialogue, we'll point out that in the second round, the therapist begins to model using verbal aikido more flexibly and fluidly by not pointing to question 3, about how the hook feels and where it shows up in her body. Pointing at the questions simply serves to reinforce the process. As clients get the approach, physically pointing to the questions can be phased out. Clients generally catch on quickly and also pick up on the cue that it's no longer necessary to point to the question, as illustrated in the rest of this dialogue.

Client: It makes me feel a bit weird (*giggling and pointing at question 2*), but I think I'm starting to get it. If I got hooked by feeling weird (*pointing at question 4*), you'd see me make a joke. But the person I want to be (*pointing at question 5*) tells you that I appreciate our work. What's important to me in saying that (*pointing at question 6*) is being authentic, and this feels good (*pointing to his chest*).

Therapist: Great! Now let's do a few rounds where we share without going through the questions sequentially. We can just point to the different parts of the matrix as we notice them coming up. I'm glad you're getting it, because you're important to me (*pointing at question 6*). My hook is that telling you this might spook you (*pointing at question 2*), and it makes me a bit tense here (*pointing at her throat*). It could make me stay superficial if I bit (*pointing at question 4*). But it's important to me to be authentic with you

	(pointing at question 6), and so is letting you know how much I admire you for sticking with this and asking that we practice in real time. Your turn.
Client:	Okay, so it feels uncomfortable *(pointing at question 2)*, and there's some anxiety here *(pointing at the top of his belly)*. That could make me dismiss your compliment *(pointing at question 4)*. But *(pointing at question 5)* I'm just going to say that I appreciate your being authentic and your help.
Therapist:	Excellent! So how was the whole thing?
Client:	Weird at first, but I think I got it.
Therapist:	It felt to me as though you felt touched by the end of it. I certainly felt touched.
Client:	Yes, that was kind of strange, wasn't it?

We realize that, like the client, you may initially find this exchange a bit strange. You may also feel that it stays pretty superficial. This is intentional and designed to illustrate how verbal aikido skills can be practiced at any emotional depth. In this exchange, the therapist chose to gradually deepen the emotional level of the conversation by sharing her own feelings regarding her client. In doing so, she's creating a context for the client to produce clinically relevant behavior—either toward moves or away moves. In this case, although Sam's request for a different way of working brought the therapist into contact with uncomfortable thoughts and feelings, she saw Sam's request as a toward move, and she sought to reinforce it by agreeing to Sam's request. As Sam engaged in verbal aikido for two, another toward move, the therapist felt closer to him and took the risk of letting Sam know how she felt. Sam responded in kind, with an additional toward move of sharing his feelings of gratitude for the work they had done.

Using Verbal Aikido for Two to Shape Interpersonal Behavior

When clients' interpersonal behaviors are particularly inflexible, this can interfere with therapy just as much as with everyday life. In such cases, verbal aikido can be quite helpful, but you'll need to slow the process way down, as these clients may not be able to identify potential toward moves. Invite the client to look at what's happening in the room step-by-step, and then ask her to identify whether she notices the next thing she does or says, including possibly remaining silent, as more of a toward move or an away move. You can prime the pump by offering to go first if it seems that would be helpful.

The following dialogue illustrates using verbal aikido for two with Rachel, a single mother who has a history of unsatisfactory intimate relationships with men, whom she invariably comes to see as self-centered. She longs for a more caring and reciprocal relationship, yet she has difficulty hearing kind words and receiving positive regard from others, especially men—including her male therapist.

Client:	I blew my top once again, and my daughter stormed out of the living room. There was no way for me to use any of what we've practiced here. I don't know if I can ever get better. By now you must despair of me.
Therapist:	That must be really hard. But you know I'm not giving up on you. I care about you.
Client:	*(Speaks in an angry tone.)* You don't mean a word of that! You only say it because it's your job.
Therapist:	I can see this is really upsetting for you. *(Rachel nods.)* Can I take a risk here?
Client:	Okay...
Therapist:	Thanks, because I'm noticing a lot of hooks in my matrix right now: fear, shame, and feeling incompetent. There's some tension in my throat. If I did bite, you would see me just move on. But the therapist I want to be would slow down and talk with you about what just happened. What's important to me in doing that is helping you work on receiving positive regard—from me and from men more generally. It feels a bit scary, and also I notice some warmth in my chest as I tell you that this is important to me. So let me ask: Is what's happening right now similar to the difficulties you experience in taking in positive regard from other men?
Client:	Yeah, I guess it's the same.
Therapist:	Would you be willing to use the verbal aikido moves like I just did?
Client:	Okay.
Therapist:	So what showed up for you when I said that I care about you?
Client:	It made me angry, and I felt like you were mocking me.
Therapist:	Okay, so as my own toward move, let me be more explicit. When I say that I care about you, what I mean—and this has nothing to do with the fact that you're paying me—is that whenever I hear that you're able to do what moves you toward who or what is important to you, I feel happy. And whenever I hear that you're stuck in away moves, I feel sad. *(Pauses.)* So how are you receiving this?
Client:	I can take in the first part, but the second part really makes me angry.
Therapist:	You mean when I say that I feel sad whenever I hear that you're stuck in away moves?
Client:	Yes. I don't believe you.

Therapist:	Okay. What hooks show up for you?
Client:	Anger, disbelief, and the thought that you're mocking me.
Therapist:	Okay. Can you show me where that shows up in your body?
Client:	Here (*pointing to her jaw*).
Therapist:	I see. And what do you do when you bite the hook?
Client:	I get angry and say what I just said.
Therapist:	Excellent. And what would the person you want to be say or do?
Client:	I don't know!
Therapist:	Would it be important to be able to respond differently?
Client:	Yes, but I don't know what else to say.
Therapist:	What would be important to you in being able to respond differently?
Client:	I don't want to turn people away.
Therapist:	And how does that feel?
Client:	Sad.
Therapist:	Yes. And where do you feel that? (*Rachel points to her chest.*) Okay, so can I suggest something else you could say when I say I care about you?
Client:	Okay.
Therapist:	How about simply saying, "Thank you"?
Client:	(*Looks down.*) Okay, then.
Therapist:	So, you know, Rachel, I care about you.
Client:	Thank you (*smirking*).
Therapist:	Well, that felt nice. I'm noticing that I feel encouraged, and that there's some more warmth here (*pointing to his chest*).
Client:	(*Smiles.*) I'm not sure I'd be able to do this out there, though.
Therapist:	Yes. That's okay. How was it doing it here?
Client:	Not as bad as I imagined.
Therapist:	You mean you noticed a hook about how bad it would be and still chose to do the toward move of saying "Thank you"?
Client:	(*Grins.*) Yes, exactly.

Using the Therapeutic Relationship in Matrix Work

In this exchange, the therapist pointed to an away move in session and offered a parallel with Rachel's difficulty in receiving positive regard from men in general. Rachel validated this interpretation, opening the door to working on it. Using verbal aikido moves, the therapist revealed his own matrix and invited Rachel to do the same. When Rachel couldn't come up with a potential toward move, the therapist made a minimalist suggestion. The reason for that minimalism is the same as that in the perspective-taking interview in chapter 6: by keeping it simple and using words that are likely to be part of the client's language, you increase the probability that the client will use them or something similar outside of session. You also reduce the chances that the client will get caught up in the words themselves.

Of course, saying thank you with a smirk that sort of belies the sentiment is not yet a workable response to an expression of positive regard. However, as compared with open hostility, it's a step in the right direction, so reinforcing it begins the process of shaping a more workable response. The therapist truly felt that Rachel's response was an improvement, so he could authentically share his positive feelings, which in turn helped Rachel respond to his further expressions of positive regard in a more effective way.

As this exchange illustrates, when clients are stuck in deeply ingrained interpersonal patterns, it can take repeated practice to help them shape behavior that's more in line with the person they want to be and that better supports the relationships they want to build. In Rachel's case, it took a few more sessions in which the therapist deliberately expressed his authentic positive regard for her before she could more openly receive what he was sharing. Subsequently, she reported being better able to both express and receive positive regard in other significant relationships.

We sometimes use another approach, which we call the two plates, in situations where it would be helpful to get a client to stop engaging in away moves in session. For example, a client may focus on stuck stories and talk in such a rapid-fire way that you can't get her to sort with the matrix. In these cases, gently ask for permission to interrupt, then present two potential moves: on one hand the current away move, and on the other a possible toward move. Then invite the client to choose which plate she wants to eat from. Make the toward move as simple as you can to maximize the chances that she'll be willing and able to engage in it.

The Matrix Session Bridging Questionnaire

We've found an approach along the lines of the FAP Session Bridging Form (Tsai et al., 2009) to be very helpful in therapeutic relationship–focused work. We've adapted and expanded the FAP Session Bridging Form to reflect our matrix orientation and invite you to use this version with your clients if you wish. (The worksheet is available for download at http://www.newharbinger.com/33605.)

The Matrix Session Bridging Questionnaire

Part A (to be completed soon after our session)

1. On a scale of 1 to 10, how much were you looking forward to our session?
_____

2. What stands out, or what did you take away from our session?

_____

_____

3. On a scale of 1 to 10, how helpful or effective was our session? _____

What was helpful? _____

_____

What wasn't helpful? _____

_____

4. On a scale of 1 to 10, how freely were you able to share with me? _____

Could I have done anything to make it easier for you to share with me? If yes, describe briefly:

_____

_____

5. On a scale of 1 to 10, how well did you feel I understood what you were thinking and feeling during our session? _____

Describe briefly: _____

_____

6. On a scale of 1 to 10, did you do your best to be engaged in the topics discussed? _____

Could I have done anything to make it easier for you to be engaged? If yes, describe briefly:

_____

_____

7. On a scale of 1 to 10, did you do your best to connect with me? _____

Could I have done anything to make it easier for you to connect with me? If yes, describe briefly:

_____

_____

8. On a scale of 1 to 10, rate your amount of toward moves in the session:

_____

9. On a scale of 1 to 10, rate your amount of away moves in the session:

_____

10. What issues came up for you in the session or with me that are similar to your problems in everyday life? Describe briefly:

_____

_____

11. What toward moves did you initiate in our session that can translate into your outside life? Describe briefly:

_____

_____

Part B (to be completed just prior to our next session)

12. What were the high points and low points of your week?

High points: _____

_____

Low points: _____

_____

13. Describe at least one toward move you engaged in. (Feel free to list more, up to one per day, on a separate piece of paper.) What did you notice?

_____

_____

14. Describe at least one away move you engaged in. (Feel free to list more, up to one per day, on a separate piece of paper.) What did you notice?

_____

_____

15. Rate whether you did your best to initiate toward moves on a scale of 1 to 10:

_____

16. What do you want to put on the agenda for our upcoming session?

_____

_____

17. On a scale of 1 to 10, how open were you in responding to these questions?

_____

18. On a scale of 1 to 10, how much are you looking forward to our upcoming session? _____

19. Anything else you'd like to add? _____

_____

As you can see, the questionnaire is divided into two sections. Part A (questions 1 through 11) assesses clients' in-session experience. Part B (questions 12 through 19) illuminates the effectiveness of the work in promoting real-life behavior change and helps set the agenda for the next session. Instruct clients to fill out part A as soon as possible after the session, while their memory of the session is still fresh, and to fill out part B just prior to your next session, responding based only on the time elapsed since your previous session.

These nineteen questions cover wide ground. Questions 1 through 3 ask clients to evaluate how much they were looking forward to the session, what stood out or what they took away from the session, and how helpful or effective the session was. Responses to these questions reveal whether your work together is broadly appetitive and effective for clients. They can also provide feedback to help you better meet your clients' needs. Make sure you respond openly and nondefensively to anything clients mention as being not helpful. In this way, you model receiving and acting on feedback. That said, your responses will also be shaped by whether what the client has written and the way she's written it seems to be more of a toward or an away move. If in doubt, or if you suspect that the client may see something differently than you do, it's best to ask for clarification.

Questions 4 through 7 focus on the quality of intimacy in the therapeutic relationship. Question 4 asks whether clients felt they could freely share with you and whether there was anything you could have done to make it easier for them to share. Question 5 asks whether you seemed to understand what was on their mind and asks for a brief description to help both of you identify what reinforces the client's sense of intimacy. Questions 6 and 7 are more active questions, inviting clients to rate whether they did their best to be engaged in the discussion and connect with you, again asking whether there was anything you could have done to make it easier for them. These active questions, in the form of "did you do your best" rather than "did you feel," help clients focus on their behavior, amidst their inner experience or external factors, while still giving them a chance to express their need for support or change on your part.

Questions 8 through 11 focus on clinically relevant behavior. Questions 8 and 9 ask clients to rate their toward and away moves in the session. Question 10 serves to identify potential CRB1 (in-session away moves that reflect their difficulties outside of session), and question 11 invites clients to identify CRB2 (in-session toward moves that they could generalize to their daily life). Having a chance to look back on the session from the perspective of identifying CRBs helps keep clients focused on in-the-moment processes and to better translate in-session progress into daily life.

Turning to part B, question 12 reviews the high and low points of the week. This helps prevent the upcoming session from getting bogged down in discussions of the "weekly news" by focusing on what stands out.

Questions 13 and 14 invite clients to record a toward move and an away move from the past week and what they noticed around these actions. These questions help clients keep on track with the main task in matrix work: noticing toward and away moves.

Question 15 is an active question that assesses clients' commitment to initiating toward moves, which can help increase their motivation to choose more toward moves.

Question 16 gives clients a chance to put items on the agenda for the upcoming session. This creates a context for working together collaboratively. You may wish to suggest other agenda items, perhaps working on one of the six steps or addressing issues clients mention in answers to other items on the questionnaire. Coming up with a collaborative agenda provides an opportunity for both therapist and client to notice toward and away moves and to practice choosing toward moves. However, given that matrix work is ultimately about helping clients choose, you may wish to let clients decide what to put on the agenda once you've made any suggestions.

Question 17 invites clients to reflect on how open they were in filling out the questionnaire. Their responses indicate their ability to relate intimately, freely sharing what they feel and think. In some cases, clients may feel so uncomfortable about sharing that they don't respond to this question openly. If you feel this may be the case, gently mention that you're having this thought and notice how the client responds. If the client doesn't validate your experience but you still have a strong sense that this is happening, she may be engaged in an away move, not seeing how others perceive her.

Question 18 asks clients to assess how much they're looking forward to the upcoming session, providing an indication of how broadly appetitive therapy is for them. Finally, question 19 gives clients a chance to add anything else they'd like to share about your work together. This is an open question that can help capture anything the other questions didn't get at. It also provides another opportunity for clients to engage in either a toward or an away move.

We've found that clients' responses to these questions contribute greatly to focusing therapy on what happens in the moment in the therapeutic relationship and that filling out the questionnaire tends to increase clients' active participation in the process both in and out of session. Still, you may feel as though nineteen questions is a lot to ask. Feel free to prune away some questions or otherwise adapt the questionnaire to better fit your style.

In our practice, we don't require any of our clients to fill it out. However, after they hear that this form helps us provide individualized treatment, over 80 percent fill it out regularly.

Taken together, these questions are a great device for tracking how clients are doing and how therapy is working for them. They help ensure that you don't miss anything happening in the therapeutic relationship that you might use to further help clients or that might be hindering their progress. An effective way to use the questionnaire is to briefly review clients' answers at the beginning of each session, perhaps after the settling-in exercise if you use that. If any responses stand out, those may guide you in choosing what to offer to work on in the session. For example, if a client felt disconnected in the previous section, you can invite her to notice how connected she's feeling in the current session and to let you know if her sense of being connected falls below a specific level. You can also invite her to discuss what both of you could do to help her feel more connected in session.

Using the Matrix to Train Perspective Taking and Empathy for Others

Because it's closely related to how the matrix is used in therapeutic relationship–focused work, we'll take this opportunity to discuss how the matrix can be used to help clients take the perspective of others they interact with. Consider a client who reports fear in response to her husband's expressions of anger at her passivity. Her therapist might ask whether she sees her husband as engaging in a toward or an away move. Her therapist can next ask what hooks the woman imagines her husband may be experiencing. When clients are able to imagine another person's perspective, they more readily feel empathy and often find new ways of relating that can foster more flexibility in the situation. Continuing with our example, the client said she would tell her husband that she understood that he felt irritated at her apparent passivity, that she's working on more clearly asserting her needs, and that she hopes he'll support her in that. She saw this as an important courage move. In the next session, she reported that she had indeed said these things to her husband and that he'd responded positively.

In some cases, the other person may not respond positively. In debriefing such situations, continue to invite clients to imagine whether the other person was on the right or left side and what the person's hooks might have been. This iterative process can be immensely helpful in bringing increased flexibility to clients' interactions. With time, perhaps the other person will begin to respond more flexibly too, and if not, that's important information in its own right.

With the most stuck clients, you can slow this process down and focus on in-session interactions. To do so, invite your client to imagine what may be showing up in your matrix and to share that with you. Then, in response, you can share authentically about what you noticed showing up. In some cases, what will have shown up for you could be pretty aversive. Maybe you've felt irritated by your client or discouraged by the slow pace of progress, or maybe you've had the thought that your client simply doesn't want to get better. In such cases, remember that authenticity is often best tempered by kindness.

CHAPTER 8

The Matrix with Children, Adolescents, and Parents

When working with children, adolescents, and their parents, we've found that the matrix can enhance the effectiveness of interventions, help young people move toward a valued life, and increase parents' engagement in providing the nurturing environment that can help their children grow to their full potential and thrive. When it comes to helping children in general, and those under twelve in particular, parents are a large part of the equation. They have a huge influence on the child's living environment and on creating and maintaining conditions that can either foster or impede their child's development. Therefore, it's important to get them to take an active role in helping their children.

This chapter gives some pointers on using the matrix when working with parents and children, including separate sections on how to adapt the approach for teenagers and for children age twelve and younger. We'll also set forth some principles for effective parenting that combine the best of behavioral approaches, emotion coaching, and insights gleaned from relational frame theory, showing you how to present these principles to parents in a way that can maximize their commitment to applying them.

Working with Parents

The stellar research in effective parenting that has taken place over the past thirty to forty years has not yet fully seeped into the culture, so many parents may still engage in less-than-optimal parenting practices simply out of ignorance. And even when parents are familiar with approaches such as positive reinforcement and validating emotions, inner obstacles can prevent them from doing what works in their parenting. The matrix can be immensely helpful in overcoming these obstacles. In this section, we'll primarily address how to get parents on board and how to adapt key matrix questions to the context of working with parents. Then we'll turn to principles for effective parenting, as those are really the heart of the matter. And as you'll see, the principles we present are also highly salient in matrix work in general.

Getting Parents On Board

When initially meeting with people who are seeking help in parenting, begin as always with the matrix, by drawing the now-familiar bisecting lines. Then ask for permission to show them a point of view that can make it easier for them to choose to do what's important in relation to their children, even in the presence of obstacles.

Using the Matrix with Parents

Once you have parents' consent, you can look at their situation through the matrix. Start by asking them who or what is important to them in coming to see you to seek help for their child. Typical answers include their child, his future, his health, his success at school, his success in friendships, preserving the family, and minimizing negative impacts on siblings. Write their responses in the lower right quadrant. Sometimes parents will (quite appropriately) say that they too are important and that they're at their wit's end. If they don't name themselves, ask them whether they're among the important people in the family. They will almost assuredly recognize that they are. Then you can add their names to the list.

Next, ask what inner stuff can show up and stand in the way of taking steps to move toward these important people and things, and write these in the lower left. With parents, there's a good chance that they'll name some outer obstacles, such as their child's oppositional behavior. If you point out that their child's behavior is an external obstacle, they may feel invalidated, especially if what brought them to you was their child's problematic behavior. So at this point, it's best not to sort between inner and outer obstacles. Just write whatever they say in the lower left quadrant. If they mention an outer obstacle, ask how that makes them feel and then write that in the lower left quadrant too.

Next, ask them what they can be seen doing to move away from or under the control of the inner obstacles listed. Typical answers include screaming, arguing, cajoling, giving up, and coming to see you. Don't hesitate to sketch a video camera outside the upper left quadrant to emphasize the focus on observable behavior.

Finally, ask what they can or could be seen doing to move toward who or what is important to them in relation to their difficulties with their child. Typical answers include coming to therapy, talking with their child's teachers, speaking to their child about the issue, and supporting each other as best they can. However, it isn't rare for parents to say they don't know what to do and that this is why they've come to see you. For an example matrix for parents, see figure 9.

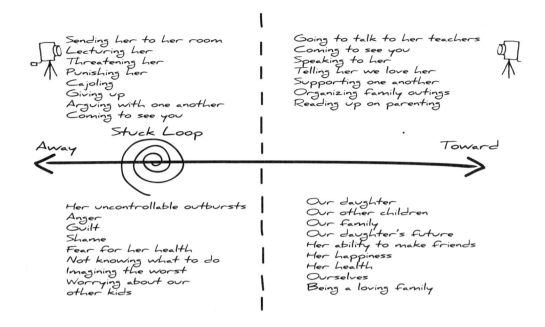

Figure 9.

Variations on the Theme

Although introducing and using the matrix with parents proceeds in much the same way as with individual clients, you'll want to make some adjustments to reflect these clients' context, as we did in the preceding section. As ever in matrix work, flexibility is key. To that end, we'll offer a few additional questions that can be helpful when working with parents (with thanks to our colleagues Timothy Gordon, Sheri Turrell, and Carlos Rivera). As you'll see, some of these questions delve into parents' family of origin, whereas others inquire about their present experience:

- What kind of parent do you want to be? What qualities in yourself matter?

- What qualities would you want to model for your child?

- What gets in the way of being the parent you want to be?

- What gets in the way of being who you want to be for your child?

- How do you handle tough emotions?

- When you were growing up, did your family members readily show emotions? If so, which ones, and how did they show them?

- When you were growing up, did you feel you were able to have and to show your emotions? What about difficult emotions like fear, anger, nervousness, or shame?

- Are there parenting habits or practices your parents used that you'd like to keep? Are there any you'd like to discard?

- What did you learn from your parents about handling difficult emotions?

- Do you find yourself trying to change your child's feelings?

- What do you feel when you're trying to change your child's emotions?

- When you look back on your childhood, do you remember doing things mostly to avoid punishment or being denied access to things you liked, or doing things mostly because you liked them and they mattered to you and receiving encouragement for doing so?

- If you could change anything in the way your parents behaved toward you or your siblings, what would you change?

Answering these questions can help parents step back from their current difficulties and consider what's important to them and what kind of an environment and relationship they want to provide for their child. Use the questions however you like. Try some of them or all of them. Offer them all at once as a questionnaire, or just use individual questions as they feel appropriate.

Promoting a Nurturing Environment

At this point, you can set the stage for sharing some key parenting principles a bit later in your work together. Explain to parents that although they probably aren't responsible for their child's difficulties, there's a great deal they can do to help and that you can share a few simple principles that help increase positive behavior in children, foster their autonomy, improve family relationships, and promote peace in the home. Explain that these principles can help create conditions optimal for their child's development—in other words, a nurturing environment.

Next, share that although these principles are simple to apply, they aren't easy to use, nor are they a magic pill. They often require a significant and permanent change in parenting practices. Point at the bottom left quadrant and tell them that, at one time or another, most parents will notice thoughts and emotions showing up and getting in the way of applying these principles consistently and that some of these thoughts and emotions may be so strong that they'll be tempted to go back to their old ways of doing things. Invite parents to share some of the things they've done as parents to move away from unwanted feelings and then ask if those feelings ever came back. Then draw the stuck loop spiral (as described in chapter 2) and explain that most parents occasionally get caught in a stuck loop, in which difficult inner experiences drive away moves, which lead, in turn, to yet more stuff showing up in the lower left quadrant. Emphasize that difficult thoughts and feelings are normal and to be expected and that the key is to not let these inner experiences drive them into a stuck loop. As you present this, you could map it out on their matrix, asking parents if they can anticipate which thoughts and emotions could show up and stand in the way of using methods that work—perhaps because they've noticed these thoughts and emotions showing up in the past. (Figure 10 illustrates a matrix diagram amended in this way.)

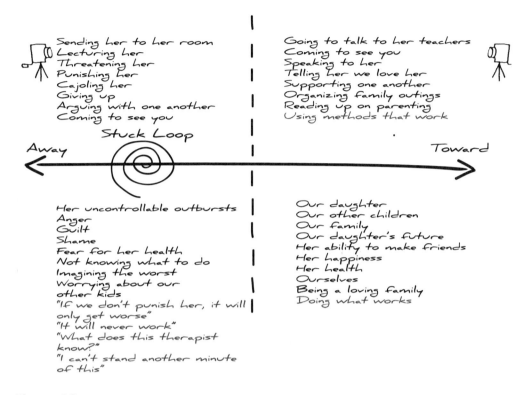

Figure 10.

Helpful Metaphors for Introducing Principles of Effective Parenting

We've found the Dancing metaphor (McCurry, 2009) useful for introducing parents to our principles for effective parenting. Here's an example of how you might present the metaphor.

Therapist: Have you ever danced or watched a professional dancer? You may know that dancing well requires a lot of practice. Professional dancers practice until the moves of the choreography become second nature. Repetition makes these movements automatic and highly efficient. In the same way, in our parenting dance we develop some automatic moves that involve interrelated ways of thinking, feeling, and acting. Although most of our dancing moves are useful, at least at times, some are automatic responses that arise from anxiety, fear, and anger. Then our dancing can move to the left-hand side of the matrix, and because it's automatic it can happen without conscious choice and even without being aware of it. Our work together is about helping you learn and practice new moves that can help you better dance with your children.

Another alternative is a jungle-related metaphor our Australian colleague Darin Cairns uses. Begin by presenting life as a jungle into which we launch our kids when we bring them into the world, then proceed along the following lines.

Therapist: As parents, we can be either guides or gatekeepers. Gatekeepers use lots of rules: "Do this," "Don't do that," and so on. Guides tell children about what they may find and invite them to notice what brings them delicious fruit and fun experiences and what leads them into dangerous situations. By using the principles I'll present shortly, you can become a more effective guide in orienting your child through the jungle of life.

Next, ask what the parents they want to be would do: Would they give up on effective parenting when the practices feel too hard and their minds tell them, "It won't work, so just give up," landing them back in their old dance moves (or turning them back into gatekeepers)? Or would they continue applying principles that are more likely to serve both their child and their relationship with him? Most parents choose the latter. You can then once again ask them who or what is important to them in being able to choose that.

Once parents have chosen to use effective parenting principles, you can introduce the principles in the next section. You can introduce them all at once, or if you prefer or it seems clients would benefit from going more slowly, you can introduce them gradually. Either way, invite clients to apply these principles and report back. This will increase the chances that they'll actually use the principles and track the results.

Some Principles of Effective Parenting and How to Present Them

A large body of research indicates that the principles of behavior analysis can be quite effective in creating nurturing environments that promote children's optimal development (Biglan, 2015). Meanwhile, John Gottman, a pioneer of relationship counseling, has advocated an approach he calls emotional coaching (1997), a specific set of parental behaviors that increase the chances that children will be able to receive the highs and lows of human emotional experience and respond to their emotions appropriately and flexibly. Combining these approaches with insights from relational frame theory, we've synthesized a set of eleven principles that serve to create and maintain a nurturing environment for children. We'll set them forth in brief list form first, parenthetically alluding to the behavioral processes at work in each. Then we'll examine each principle more closely, give pointers on how to present it, and address how that principle plays out more generally in therapeutic work with clients.

1. Validate unconditionally all of your child's thoughts, feelings, and emotions, establishing that all inner experience is okay. (This weakens the control of aversive inner experience over behavior.)

2. Invite your child to notice, through experience, that some behavior is workable and some is not. (This prompts noticing workability.)

3. Water what you want to see grow, using positive reinforcement in your interactions with your children. (This employs appetitive control to broaden behavioral repertoire.)

4. Consistently speak in terms of what you want your child to do and the potential rewards, rather than what you don't want him to do and the likely punishment. (Consistent use of appetitive verbal rules makes parents predictable and trustworthy guides).

5. When you give your child instructions, describe some of what might happen and invite him to notice what happens when he does or doesn't follow the instructions. (This engages tracking to promote flexibly following helpful rules.)

6. Ask kindly and clearly and provide choices. (This sets up appetitive antecedents for the target behavior, increasing the likelihood of the child engaging in the behavior.)

7. Split tasks in smaller chunks and, when this can be useful, offer to start the task with your child. (This uses shaping to develop the desired behavior.)

8. When asking for a low-probability behavior, first ask for a high-probability behavior. (This increases the chances of getting behavior that can then be reinforced in its own right.)

9. When your child engages in good behavior, praise both the behavior and the child himself. When your child engages in bad behavior, stick to behavior-based talk. (This promotes inner motivation, a healthy sense of self, and a sense that unworkable behavior can be changed.)

10. Let the consequences do the talking; in other words, demonstrate empathy when your child meets aversive consequences—even when you are the person delivering the consequences. (This is a nurturing way of using contingencies to extinguish undesired behaviors.)

11. Use moments when your child is experiencing difficult emotions as opportunities to move toward connection before moving to problem solving. (This trains children to relate intimately by encouraging them to connect by sharing what they feel.)

Clearly, these principles go beyond matrix work, so in this chapter we'll just outline how you can present them to parents and give a rationale for following them. For a fuller treatment of some of these principles, refer to *Parent Management Training* (Kazdin, 2005); for parents, you can recommend that they read *The Everyday Parenting Toolkit*, by Alan Kazdin and Carlo Rotella (2013), or *The Joy of Parenting*, by Lisa Coyne and Amy Murrell (2009). Another good resource is John Gottman's *The Heart of Parenting: Raising an Emotionally Intelligent Child* (1997). Before we dive into the principles, one final note: Although it's a bit off topic for this chapter, for each of the following principles, we'll also briefly describe its broader role in enhancing the effectiveness of therapy with any client.

1. Validate all thoughts, feelings, and emotions

This principle is at the heart of much of the matrix work in step 3, exploring the effectiveness of control efforts in the inner world versus the outer world. You can present it to parents in much the same way as in chapter 3. Once parents have experienced the futility of attempting to control their inner experience, they may be more open to another approach: unconditionally validating everything their child feels or thinks. This can be a good time to ask parents how they habitually respond to their own difficult thoughts and emotions and how they habitually respond to those of their child.

In matrix work, and in ACT more generally, unconditionally validating all inner experience is essential. Because the matrix trains noticing, it effectively teaches people to make room for all inner experience. However, the therapist's stance is crucial in promoting acceptance of inner experience, and the validation strategies in chapter 4 are invaluable in this regard. Verbal aikido and self-compassion work can also promote acceptance of inner experience.

2. Invite your child to notice that some behavior is workable and some is not

Make it clear to parents that validating thoughts and emotions doesn't mean giving children a license to behave in inappropriate or unworkable ways. Far from it. Although parents and children alike have little control over their thoughts and emotions, we all have much greater control over our behavior, including what we say. Part of the role of parents is to give children a chance to experience which behaviors work and which don't. So an important part of the job of parenting is to set limits and establish consequences for unworkable behavior—and, of course, rewards for good behavior.

More broadly, it's much harder to not do something than to learn to do something else. For example, it's much harder to stop swearing than to learn how to express what the problem is. When working for behavior change, a first step is to describe precisely what the desired, observable behavior would look like, rather than what it shouldn't look like.

Another way to notice workability is by sorting with the matrix. When working with clients, inviting them to notice workability is key, as is inviting them to identify toward moves, rather than fighting to repress away moves.

3. Water what you want to see grow

Once parents are on board with promoting new behavior, introduce positive reinforcement as the most effective tool for change. Explain that all behavior is maintained by the consequences it receives. For humans, receiving attention from others is highly reinforcing—so much so that problematic behavior can be maintained simply by receiving negative attention from parents, peers, or teachers. Invite parents to turn their attention toward what their child is doing right and catch him "being good." Then outline the three components of effective reinforcement: briefly describing the behavior to their child, using an enthusiastic tone in doing so, and making affectionate physical contact. You might also mention that tone and physical contact should be adapted depending on the child's age. With toddlers, high fives and enthusiastic oohs and aahs work well, whereas with teenagers, a calm and positive tone and a light brush of the arm might work better. It can be challenging for parents to remember all three elements, so don't hesitate to role-play them with parents until they've got it down.

More generally, matrix work is about reinforcing a specific behavior: noticing with the matrix. As discussed in chapter 7, on therapeutic relationship–focused work, positive reinforcement can also be used to shape particular interpersonal behaviors. Whatever the intervention, matrix practitioners always seek to make matrix work inherently reinforcing so that clients will be more likely to continue engaging with the matrix.

4. Consistently speak in terms of what you want your child to do and the potential rewards

When it comes to their kids, parents' attention is naturally drawn to avoiding potential dangers and solving problems. This naturally leads to emphasizing don'ts over dos. Whether the danger is immediate, as in "Don't touch the stove!" or more long-term, as in "Don't eat so much sugar or your teeth will rot," negative commands and rules often predominate. The problem is that overusing these commands and rules outside of immediate physical emergencies tends to reinforce away moves, and this can result in kids ending up in stuck loops at the cost of moving toward a valued life. So encourage parents to use positively worded rules; for example, "Please help with the dishes and then you can play on the computer," rather than "If you don't help with the dishes, you won't be allowed to use the computer."

Matrix work also benefits from devoting attention to providing clients with appetitive rules. So aim for statements that emphasize appetitive control, such as "By trying out new behaviors, people can move toward who or what is important." Do your best to steer clear of formulations that rely on aversive control, such as "If you don't start doing this, you'll never live a valued life."

5. When you give your child instructions, describe some of what might happen and encourage tracking

The more children notice the broader consequences of their behavior, the more flexible and attuned to their environment they become. Although it can be tempting for stressed-out and overworked parents to tell their kids to follow instructions "because I told you so," this sows the seeds of rebellion and leads to coercive and threatening relationships. Simply put, it makes kids move away from their parents—something you can emphasize by asking parents for examples of times when that might have happened. Another nefarious side effect of saying things like "because I told you so" is that it can lead kids to pay more attention to the effects of their behavior on the person who gave the instructions than on what else happens, thereby narrowing their attention to pliance and counterpliance and restricting their flexibility. (For a fuller discussion of pliance and counterpliance, refer back to chapter 5.)

Advise parents to find ways to encourage their child to notice what he experiences when he does something, even when they feel tempted to simply tell him what to do. For example, a parent might say, "Put on your winter gloves and see if you can notice whether your hands stay warm and you can play in the snow longer." Be clear that this is about inviting their child to notice what happens in fairly close temporal proximity to a behavior, not about lecturing on the distant future perils and rewards of a given behavior (for example, "Practice writing the letter A and notice that you can get into an Ivy League college"). A fun way to get parents into tracking is to invite them to notice, through the lens of the matrix, what happens in their interactions with their child. For example, how does their use (or nonuse) of effective parenting principles affect their interactions? In this way, they too get to notice consequences, rather than simply submitting to the rules you give them or reacting to stuff on the left-hand side of their matrix.

This principle is about promoting flexible tracking—noticing the consequences of one's behavior beyond simply whether one has followed a particular rule or not. As discussed in chapters 2 and 3, using the matrix promotes flexible tracking of important aspects of our context and experience. The same principle is at work in the basic verbal aikido moves, in which clients are invited to notice their inner experience, their behavior, and their five-senses experience, which can extend to what happened both before and after a particular behavior.

6. Ask kindly and provide choices

An extremely effective way of promoting a desired behavior is to provide appetitive antecedents. And not surprisingly, kindness tends to be highly appetitive, with requested behavior being more likely after asking nicely than asking sternly or sarcastically. If need be, explain to parents that if their tone is unpleasant when asking their child to help with chores, for example, it's more likely that their child won't comply. Another possibility is that their child will comply, but only to escape the aversive nature of the request, in which case complying is an away move that creates distance in the relationship. It can be especially easy to forget this simple step of asking nicely when dealing with a recalcitrant teenager. Of course, asking kindly goes hand in hand with asking clearly and firmly, and it can work wonders in even the most entrenched family difficulties.

Sometimes children ignore requests or mock them. For children who tend to ignore requests, invite parents to simply restate their instructions and then ask their child to state his understanding of the request, the (preferably) appetitive consequences of complying, and (as rarely as possible) the aversive consequences of not complying. For children who tend to respond with sarcasm, encourage parents to ignore their child's tone and respond only to the elements of his answer that reflect the request. Also acknowledge that it's very difficult to ignore a child's sarcasm. With parents in this situation, explore the alternative: becoming a gatekeeper—someone their child will want to move away from. Invite parents to ignore mocking, sarcasm, and other such behavior and to reinforce desired behavior as much as feasible.

With parents who are really struggling, it can be helpful to practice this skill in session. Be clear, however, that this principle, like all the others, is probabilistic. None have a 100 percent success rate; they simply make particular behaviors and outcomes more or less probable. The fact that results are probabilistic is actually good news for parents, as it means they don't have to seek perfection and stick to these principles 100 percent of the time; as long as they adhere to them about 70 to 80 percent of the time, they're likely to get good results.

Parents can leverage the power of this approach by offering choices. For example, asking a child if he wants to first wash his hands and then put away his toys or first put away his toys and then wash his hands is more likely to get him to both wash his hands and put away his toys than asking him to do both without framing it as a choice. When presenting this principle to parents, be sure to mention that both of the choices they offer should be acceptable to them. You might exemplify this point by saying something like, "If you ask your child to choose between putting away his toys and you putting them away, be prepared to put them away yourself!" As a rationale for using this strategy, explain that children who have experience in making choices are more likely to choose wisely as they grow up and to prefer people and jobs in which they have a choice in life. Simply ask parents what they would choose for their child if they could: a life with choices or a life without them?

Of course, offering choices is sometimes useful and sometimes less effective. Invite parents to notice situations where it doesn't work. In such cases, they can return to simply stating the request kindly and clearly.

More generally, as a matrix practitioner it is your mission to be kind, warm, and genuine—in other words, to provide an appetitive interpersonal context in which clients are more likely to try new behaviors. And working with the matrix is deliberately about promoting choice. When clients start noticing that they have a choice, they're more likely to choose toward moves. This makes it all the more important to avoid giving clients the impression that your aim is to make them engage in toward moves, instead being clear that your aim is to help them broaden their choices.

7. Split tasks into smaller chunks and, if necessary, offer to start difficult tasks with your child

Sometimes children don't engage in a behavior parents ask for because it's too complex. In this case, it's helpful to divide the task into smaller bites. If parents want their child to get dressed on his own, a task that requires a lot of behaviors, they can start by asking him to choose his clothes for the day from a number of season-appropriate options. Next, they can ask him to take off his pajamas, then to put on his underwear, then to put on his shirt, and so on.

When trying out complex, new, or low-probability behaviors, parents can also get the ball rolling by starting the task with their child. For example, if they're trying to get their child to put away his toys, they can offer to start with him. When used in combination with the other principles, this can be a helpful last resort with children who won't do particular tasks.

Any time you begin matrix work with new clients, you take this approach, splitting the task of noticing with the matrix into easily digestible bites as you invite them to first notice the difference between toward and away moves, then the distinction between five-senses experience and inner experience, and so on. As you've learned, we advocate slowing down any time clients are having difficulty understanding what you're presenting or practicing a particular skill, and, if needed, engaging in the task with clients.

8. When asking for a low-probability behavior, first ask for a high-probability behavior

If parents know their child is unlikely to comply with a request for a particular behavior, they can try first asking for a behavior he engages in readily. For example, if their child readily gives hugs but resists putting on his pajamas, they might try asking for a hug first and then asking him to put on his pajamas. See if you can help parents identify some high-probability behaviors they can ask for before requesting low-probability behaviors from their child. Then invite them to provide many opportunities for the more probable behavior. For example, say goofing around and joking are highly probable, whereas doing difficult math homework is less probable. Before starting a difficult math session, a parent could joke around with his child for a while and then invite him to have a snack together, before finally turning to the math session.

This principle translates directly into matrix work and is extremely effective with clients who are well and truly stuck. The more clients are stuck, the harder it will be for them to choose to engage in toward moves out of session. However, after some practice in sorting with the matrix, the act of sorting may become more probable than engaging in outward toward moves. Then you can ask such clients to practice sorting in stuck situations (by now a relatively high-probability behavior) before choosing toward moves and, ultimately, engaging in those moves.

9. Orient your child toward sources of inner reinforcement for good behavior

When children engage in good behavior, parents naturally feel proud and willingly reinforce that behavior. While this is, of course, important, it's just as important to sow the seeds of internal reinforcement so children can be reinforced by what they do, rather than solely by rule givers expressing how happy they are with the behavior. For example, if a child has succeeded at taking a spin on his bike without his mom holding the bike, his mom could say, "You must be so proud of yourself," rather than "Mommy is so proud of you." Similarly, invite parents to frame their child's good behavior in terms of positive self-qualities. For example, if a child shares his Halloween candy with his sister, they can reinforce this by saying, "That was a very generous thing you did; you shared your candy," rather than "I'm so pleased that you shared your candy."

Inversely, and this is often hard for parents to do, when children engage in unworkable or disruptive behavior, it's important to keep the focus on the behavior, rather than the child's self. For example, they could say, "You stole your sister's candy; that's not something we want you to do," rather than denigrating the child himself with a statement like "You thief! You stole your sister's candy knowing full well that it's wrong to steal." Because children are so quick to derive a sense of self from their feelings and behavior, parents need to contribute to their budding self-conceptualization in nurturing and positive ways.

In broader clinical practice, most clients' sense of self is probably already entrenched as a function of earlier life experiences. This makes it all the more important to help them see their toward moves for what they are: something they can be proud of choosing, without insisting they should see it your way. Similarly, don't hesitate to tell them that they're courageous when they step outside of their comfort zone. And when looking at their difficulties, share that, from your perspective, what gets them stuck is away moves, not some defective aspect of who they are deep down.

10. Let the consequences do the talking

Empathy is key to a nurturing environment, and in many contexts, parents readily express empathy when their children encounter aversive consequences. This can be harder for parents to do when they've tried to educate their child about these consequences, and even harder when parents themselves have established the consequences for a particular behavior. When the consequences were established or discussed in advance, parents may default to lecturing (or worse) and more seldom show empathy for how it feels to their child to meet these consequences. This approach is generally doomed to be ineffective, as children tend to respond poorly to feeling that they are being chastised. Invite parents to notice when they engage in lecturing. It's much more effective to empathize and let the consequences do the talking.

Parents may benefit from an example. Choose something age-appropriate. If their child is in middle school, you might offer the example of telling their child, "If you do your homework, you can watch television for an hour." If he then fails to do his homework, rather than saying something like "I told you so, but you never listen," they could say, "I know it's hard, and I'm sorry that you can't watch television because you didn't do your homework. I like letting you watch television, and I hope you'll choose to do your homework tomorrow." Also cover the eventuality that their child may argue, and suggest that they default to a simple statement like "I know it's hard. Let's talk about this later." With parents of younger children, it may be best to orient them toward principle 11 and help them learn how to validate their child when he's experiencing negative emotions.

In matrix work, you'll seldom deliver aversive consequences in the way parents sometimes have to. However, clients often experience the aversive consequences of choosing to engage in away moves over toward moves. For that matter, they may experience aversive consequences even when engaging in toward moves. In all cases, validate how hard it is to experience these consequences and refrain from lecturing.

11. Use moments when your child is experiencing difficult emotions as opportunities to connect

When children experience strong negative emotions, parents naturally see this as a problem to solve. Parents don't like to see their child suffer or express anger toward them. In those situations, it's natural for parents to go straight into problem-solving mode or even to move away if their child's emotional state makes them feel bad or defective. However, this sends the message that emotions are bad, possibly dangerous, or a problem to be solved or moved away from—the very process that gets people caught in stuck loops.

A better approach is for parents to recognize that these moments provide precious opportunities to connect with their child and help him receive and name his emotions. Being validated in this way also helps children gradually learn how to self-validate. This is the heart of John Gottman's emotion coaching approach (1997), which he presents as five discrete steps:

1. Notice your child's emotions.

2. Recognize strong negative emotions as an opportunity to connect with your child and engage in emotion coaching.

3. Listen with empathy, reflecting and validating your child's feelings.

4. Help your child name the emotion he's feeling.

5. When you feel you've connected with your child's emotions, you can turn to problem solving, while also maintaining clear limits on which behaviors are possible.

This is a fairly involved process, and parents will need to practice the approach in order to use it naturally and effectively. You can refer parents to Gottman's book, though in most cases you may be able to train them to use these steps effectively. In the meanwhile, they will probably benefit from a concrete example. Here's one way you might present it.

Therapist: Imagine that your four-year-old, Thomas, doesn't want to get dressed to go to the park and starts crying and throwing a tantrum. The first step would be to recognize what he's feeling and thinking. You might say something like "You don't want to put on your coat, and you're feeling sad and angry." For the second step, recognizing and taking advantage of a teaching moment, move toward him with a warm and open manner. Squat down at his level and say something like "Let's talk about it." For the third step, listening with empathy, ask him what's going on and reflect what he says: "You want to keep playing with your blocks and don't want to go outside now. I understand that. When I want to do something and can't, I also feel angry. You want to stay here. It's okay to want that and to feel sad and angry." Then, for the fourth step, try to help him find words to express what he's feeling. In this case, you might say, "You're sad and you want to stay home. Is that right? And you're angry because I'm taking you to the park." Only move to the fifth step after you've connected with your child. You'll notice that you have when your child validates your formulation. Moving to the next step, set clear limits as you engage in problem solving. For example, you might say, "Let's see what we can do. We are going to the park. First we can talk a little bit, and then you can choose which coat you want to wear. And when we come back you can play with your blocks again."

Of course, doing matrix work with adults looks quite different than dealing with an irate toddler! That said, similar principles do apply. Before inviting clients to consider any kind of solution, express empathy for what they're experiencing. Then help them connect with what they're feeling and give them a chance to name their emotions, coaching them if need be. If you like, or if it seems helpful, use verbal aikido to help them notice where these feelings show up physically. Only after engaging them in the first four steps would you invite them to consider the choices they have and what they may wish to do other than engaging in away moves and potentially getting caught in a stuck loop.

Adapting the Matrix for Teenagers

Now we turn to working directly with children. We'll start with teenagers because, with younger children, there's a good chance that you'll be working primarily with the parents rather than the child. In our experience, teenagers typically move through the six steps in part 1 faster than adults. This may come from the fact that their stuck loops aren't so entrenched, allowing them to get unstuck faster. In general, the work proceeds as outlined in part 1. However, certain modifications can help, so we'll describe the adaptations here.

Keeping It Simple

Teenagers are notorious for not easily engaging in long, abstract discussions with adults. While asking open-ended questions is often recommended in working with adults, if you do this with teenagers in a therapy context, you risk receiving monosyllabic answers. It's often more effective to engage teens in activities and then debrief their experience than to ask them questions, even ACT-inspired questions such as what they value in life.

We've found that teenagers easily adopt the matrix point of view, even if they're unable to fill in many details. Remember that matrix work isn't about having people name everybody and everything that's important to them, notice all of their inner obstacles, or describe all of their away and toward moves; it's about looking through the point of view. With teens, keep the focus on taking a look through the point of view and give them a sense that they're succeeding. A sparse matrix works just as well as a detailed one.

Also, be sure to ask "Who is important?" first. If you ask "What's important to you?" first, you're more likely to get vague answers or statements like "I don't know." That said, some teens will also have difficulty stating who is important. If they struggle to come up with material for the lower right quadrant, you might make a few suggestions. Just be sure to offer them as examples, making it clear you don't claim to know what's going on for the client. Then stick to examples that are common for teens and that show up often in daily life, such as friends, music, family relationships, sports, movies or TV series, or even school.

Keeping It Visual

When working with teens, it's a good idea to keep things visual by referring back to the matrix diagram repeatedly. Use drawings and graphics throughout all six steps. If possible, draw little cartoons and illustrations yourself. The illustrated stuck matrix presented in figure 11 (available for download at http://www.newharbinger.com/33605)

can be a great tool for helping teens connect directly to the functions of behaviors without getting stuck due to an initial inability to describe content.

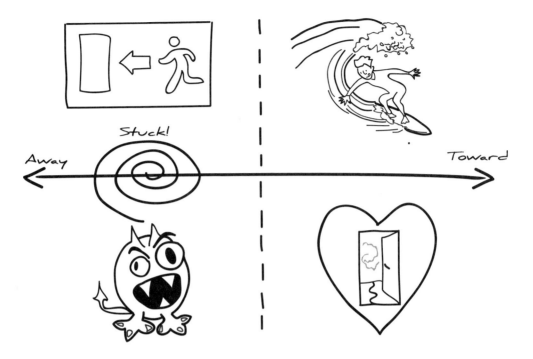

Figure 11.

We have developed two cartoon characters, called Spiky and Flexi, to capture the distinction between away and toward moves. Although originally created for adult work (Schoendorff, Grand, & Bolduc, 2011), they are very helpful in working with teenagers. These characters can be mapped onto the matrix, as in figure 12 (available for download at http://www.newharbinger.com/33605). Here's how you can present them.

Therapist: So we can be like either of these characters, Spiky and Flexi. Spiky experiences uncomfortable or painful stuff, represented by those spikes in the lower left. In response to that, he engages in away moves. The thing is, those often produce spikes out there in the world of the five senses. When Spiky gets caught up in away moves, he doesn't engage in many toward moves. Plus, because of all those spikes, he has a hard time contacting who or what is important to him. The important stuff may even become painful, in which case Spiky might feel as though nothing is important in an attempt to not experience that pain.

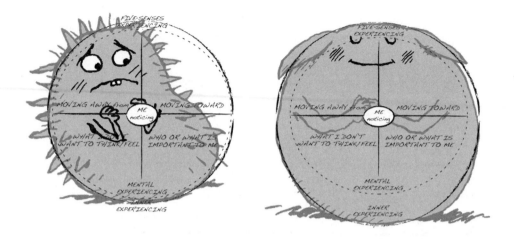

Figure 12.

One result of all of this is that Spiky contracts, shrinking away from painful experience. Explain that it's natural to contract when uncomfortable or painful stuff shows up. Another way to present this visually is to show the client your own typical bodily posture when painful stuff shows up. Then ask him to show you how he holds his body when this stuff shows up. If need be, you can prompt with a question: "Are your chest and shoulders wide open and your head held high, or are your shoulders contracted, chest sunk in, and head down?"

Continuing with Spiky, you might share that he appears spiky to others, which may make them move away from him. In addition, spiky people and spiky life events can easily get entangled in his spikes. Another issue is that responding in a spiky way can make others turn spiky. Be sure to mention that everybody gets spiky from time to time. The problem is, when we do this too often, we tend to get stuck and rarely have fun.

Then offer an alternative: that Spiky can turn into Flexi. How? Instead of trying to not feel what he doesn't want to feel and engaging in away moves, he makes space for what shows up. As Flexi, he pauses to consider which hooks are showing up, what the person he wants to be would do, and who or what is important to him in the situation. Then he chooses what he does. Flexi is a master of verbal aikido.

Practicing Verbal Aikido

The verbal aikido approach outlined in chapter 4 works well with most teens. And once they get it, they can apply it to many stuck situations at home, at school, or with peers. The metaphor of aikido often appeals to teenagers because it conveys both an active, "fighting" stance and the goal of peace and harmony. Despite the seeming contrast, both are often appetitive to teenagers.

Teenagers often struggle with many aspects of emotional experience. They don't always have the skills to recognize and name what they're feeling, and many feel overwhelmed and out of control in the face of strong emotions. The inner experience layer of the Verbal Aikido Worksheet, as described in chapter 4, can be very useful in helping them locate and name what they feel. You can use that part of the worksheet for a deliberate exercise in naming and locating feelings, gently coaching teenage clients in naming what they feel when they don't seem to have the words they need. If you do this, be sure to take the stance of holding your words and emotion labels lightly, as they will only be useful if the client recognizes them and makes them his own. When used in this way, verbal aikido can be a highly effective first step in helping teens develop the capacity to live with their feelings and emotions.

Presenting Home Practice

Some teenagers respond well to rules and homework, but many don't. So when inviting them to engage in home practice, it's especially important to let them know they don't have to do the exercises as long as they notice if they do them or if they don't. This can be a surprisingly effective way to create some space in which they feel free to choose to do them. You can say something like "This isn't school. It's not about homework, and even less about having to do something or not do something. It's about you, what is or could be important to you, and how you can more easily choose to do what you really want to do."

Being Authentic and Emphasizing Validation

When working with teenagers, whose "fakeness detectors" can be highly sensitive, authenticity is your best ally. Teens rarely react well to people who tell them what to do or who don't practice what they preach. Don't hesitate to share your own matrix. However, as you do so, take care not to seem to engage in one-upmanship or share in a way that could invalidate the teen's experience and feelings. Teenagers may appreciate hearing how you struggled as a youth, yet hearing how you overcame your difficulties may lead them to judge themselves as hopeless if they haven't yet experienced overcoming their own difficulties.

Also keep in mind that teenagers are faced with a host of difficult challenges that seem to rush at them from all directions. Their bodies are changing quickly and sometimes painfully. Their social circles are evolving rapidly. They are biologically wired to seek new environments and experiences, sometimes at the expense of safety and social norms. They're often subjected to intense peer pressure, and they face an ever-present risk of hurtful social rejection. They are subject to increasing performance pressures and the specter of seemingly decisive life choices, such as choosing a career path, moving away from the family nest, and finding a partner. These are among the highest sources of stress humans can face, and teenagers have to face them all—at a time when most of them aren't yet fully equipped to make informed choices. Maintaining an active awareness of the scale of these challenges can inform your verbal aikido stance and help you bring deep empathy and validation to the work.

Also bear in mind that teens are often subject to harsh judgments from their peers and from themselves. The Mother Cat Exercise in step 5 can be particularly effective for helping them develop more self-compassion. One reason this exercise works so well with teens is that many of them have a clear notion of how they'd like to be validated and supported by their parents, making it easy for them to access qualities of "the mother cat they want to be."

Using the Perspective-Taking Interview

The perspective-taking interview described in chapter 6 is a very powerful tool for working with teens. In this stage of their lives, they're often trying out different behaviors in different contexts. The perspective-taking interview can help them practice new behaviors in a number of different contexts: at home with family, at school, among their peers, and so on. When you invite them to choose situations to practice with, they're likely to zero in on whatever is currently most sticky for them.

Watching for Pliance and Counterpliance

Because of the many pressures they face and due to their verbal and social development, children, and teens in particular, are extremely sensitive to pressure and demands. Whenever you ask them a question, chances are their mind will try to figure out what answer you want to hear. It is thus all the more important to remember that, once you orient them to the matrix, you aren't invested in a particular answer. Teens will try to second-guess you. If you feel this is happening, you can say something along the following lines.

Therapist: Right now, my mind is telling me that maybe your mind is telling you I'd like you to sort this as a toward move [or an away move, as appropriate]. Is it just my mind, or is yours in on this too? If so, I want you to know that only you can notice where this goes in your matrix. What my mind might think or want has nothing to do with it.

When you interact in this way, you deliberately undermine both pliance and counterpliance, potentially creating a context more favorable to choosing freely and then flexibly tracking the results.

Adapting the Matrix for Children Twelve and Under

Working with children twelve and under differs from working with other clients in many ways. First, there is the fact that in most cases it's best to involve the parents, as they have a large measure of control over many of the conditions that can help or hinder the child's development. So in most cases you'll want to get parents on board and actively involved in creating a nurturing home environment, or at least in reducing unhelpful interpersonal stuck loops. This may mean that direct work with the child is less important, especially if the child's difficulties are externalized, showing up as inappropriate behaviors at home, at school, or with peers. These are some of the reasons we chose to begin this chapter by addressing how to work with parents.

All of that said, in many cases you may want to work directly with the child, even as you work with the parents. And in some cases, it might not be possible to secure parent or caregiver cooperation in the work beyond bringing the child to you. Working directly with children can also be useful when the child's difficulties are more internalized, such as anxiety or depression, as well as with some externalized problems related to emotion regulation, such as separation anxiety and explosive anger.

Keeping It Simple

The ability to talk about inner experience and identify values in abstract terms is generally even less developed in younger children than it is in teenagers. They haven't yet had the time and experience necessary to learn to name their inner experience precisely and make clear life choices. So when working with children, the less you rely on a sophisticated verbal repertoire, the more likely you are to connect with them. Because the matrix is an inherently simple tool, it can help keep you on track.

You may wish to change up the vocabulary for various aspects of the matrix, especially for quite young children. For example, instead of using "inner obstacles" to refer to content in the lower left quadrant, you might term this "That scary or angry Mr. Yucky inside." For the bottom right quadrant, you might talk about "who and what you really love." For the top left, you could say "what you feel forced to do," and for the top right, "what you'd really want to do for who and what you love."

Also note that young children often express who or what is important to them in terms of actions rather than by more abstractly naming who or what is important to them. For example, a child might say he loves playing with friends rather than saying friendship is important, or that he loves going to movies with his dad rather than saying his dad is important. That's fine. Just write these actions and the people they want to do them with in the lower right quadrant, and in the upper right list specific instances when they engaged in those actions or plan to.

Keeping It Visual and Fun

When working the matrix with younger children, use visual tools wherever possible and point first and foremost to actions. Including an image of a video camera above the horizontal line generally suffices to help them make the distinction between five-senses and inner experience. You might also want to use images to encapsulate what each quadrant gets at. For example, a monster for the lower left quadrant, an emergency exit sign for the upper left, a heart for the lower right, and a snail coming out of its shell or a surfer for the upper right. You can draw those images yourself or use the stuck matrix diagram from earlier in this chapter.

We've found it helpful to use a cardboard matrix and pictures or photos of activities, emotions, and situations relevant to the child we're working with, incorporating the realms of family, school, and peer situations as appropriate. Children will readily start sorting pictures in the matrix. The more playful you make it, the easier it will be to engage kids in sorting. When talking about a difficult situation, it can be effective to write the content of what the child is experiencing on index cards, and then hand the cards to the child and invite him to place them on the cardboard matrix wherever they seem to belong.

Another engaging way to keep it visual is to invite children (and teens) to draw portraits, figurative or abstract, of various elements of their matrix. This works especially well with inner obstacles, as it promotes noticing and defusing from difficult inner experiences. This is a great alternative to trying to get kids to talk about things for which they don't have words, and because it's fun, it makes matrix work appealing. In a blank bound book, both you and the child could draw the matrix and diverse aspects of the work, such as what the child likes to do, whom he likes to do it with, the stuff inside that he doesn't like, and so on. He can then keep the book for future reference and continue drawing matrices and other aspects of his experience after you've finished working together.

Being Transparent

Children learn a lot through modeling. You can promote that by transparently showing your own inner processes and your own sorting onto the matrix. Offering a running commentary on what's going on in your matrix, possibly in the voice of a TV sports commentator, can be a fun and effective way to do this. Here's an example of what a therapist told Paul, a ten-year-old client, while making a pretend microphone with his hand.

Therapist: So, dear viewers, right now I'm noticing a fear of being ridiculous showing up on the playing field right there (*pointing at the bottom left quadrant*). If I did bite that hook, you would see me kick the ball to the top left while talking in a very serious tone and trying to look professional (*pointing at the top left quadrant*). But the player I want to be kicks the ball to the top right by showing Paul how things are in my matrix (*pointing at the top right quadrant*). I do that because it's important to me to show Paul that we're in the same boat (*pointing at the bottom right quadrant*). And now, dear viewers, let me hand the microphone over to Paul for the next play.

Working with the Six Steps

When working with younger children, you can use all six steps of the basic matrix approach outlined in part 1 of the book. You'll just need to make age-appropriate adjustments, including simplifying some of the exercises. The Hooks metaphor generally works well with kids, though adding the catch-and-release element would probably make it too complex. A fun approach is to use a magnetic fishing game, writing difficult inner experiences like "fear," "anger," "sadness," and "worry" on the fishes. Then, when you ask what kids do next after catching a particular fish, you can write their response on a sticky note and put it on the fishing rod.

At first, you may want to keep verbal aikido as simple as possible when working with young kids, not introducing the experience layer and "where in your body" questions until they are able to use the other moves. This streamlines the approach and ensures that it isn't complex and overwhelming at first.

Further Exercises for Children

When doing matrix work with young children, you can keep it simple, experiential, and fun—and therefore more effective—by using games, toys, and engaging activities. We've found that noticing practice, in particular, lends itself to fun interactive games. Here are a few such exercises, some of which we've developed with the helpful input of our Argentinian colleague Yanina Alladio. Most of these exercises can be done with kids and their parents, offering a wonderful opportunity for them to create a new dance between them.

The Stuck Loop Car

A fun way to illustrate stuck loops is to use a cardboard matrix and toy cars. Taxis or buses are best, as they typically have a prechosen destination. Have a few of these on hand so the child can choose one. Then, as you ask questions about a difficult inner experience (say anger) and what he does next (such as hitting), drive the car in a semi-circle from lower left to upper left. Stop to ask if the inner experience came back, and if it did, drive the car back down to the lower left—and so on for a few rounds. Next, validate the child's experience by saying you understand and the behavior makes sense in its way. Then ask, "And when do you get to drive your car toward what you really want to do?" As you do so, roll the car from the lower left quadrant to the upper right. You can keep using the car as you discuss other things, asking the child to drive the car to wherever he feels he is in the conversation.

The Differences Detective

The differences detective is a game that helps promote noticing the difference between five-senses and inner experience. Before conducting this exercise, you'll need to prepare a box containing objects clients can see, hear, smell, taste, and touch. To introduce the game, invite the child to play detectives. Ask him to spend a few minutes silently observing the objects, just like detectives do. Then close the box and ask him to imagine the sight, sound, smell, taste, and touch of the objects and to name each one in turn. Finally, invite him to open his eyes and, like a detective, notice the difference between actually seeing, hearing, smelling, tasting, and touching each object and imagining doing that when the box was closed.

The Matrix Explorer

For this game, you'll need a set of index cards, each specifying a different age-appropriate noticing activity. We introduce this game using the vertical line of the matrix, explaining that the aim is to be an explorer, discovering things in the world of the five senses and in the inner world. Then we set a timer for a brief amount of time, say ten seconds, and pass the set of cards around between the child, his parents, and the therapist until the timer rings. When it does, whoever is holding the deck draws a card and engages in the activity described. Here are some sample activities:

- Listening to the sounds in the room for thirty seconds

- Closing your eyes and picturing objects in the room.

- Eating a piece of fruit or candy as if you were an alien who had never tasted it before

- Walking around the room as if you were walking on clouds

- Closing your eyes and imagining the smell and taste of your favorite fruit

- Breathing as if you were walking, then as if you were running, then as if you were eating, and describing the difference

- Doing Darth Vader breathing (see McCurry, 2009)

Sorting a Story

Invite the child to choose one of his favorite stories, whether from a book, a movie, a TV show, a comic book, or some other story. The key is that the story be age appropriate, which you can ensure by asking the child to choose it. This will also help him be more engaged in the game and committed to it. Then invite the child to imagine the emotions, thoughts, and body sensations of the main character or whichever character the child identifies with and sort them in the matrix. Next invite the child to tell any story he wishes about the character in the story while sorting thoughts, emotions, and behaviors onto the matrix. Once the sorting is over, invite the child to identify the inner obstacle that's most familiar to him in that story and to tell you what he usually does when it shows up and what he would like to be able to do.

Matrix Boxes

For this exercise you'll need index cards and four boxes a bit larger than the cards. The boxes will stand in place of the quadrants of the matrix, so label them in a way that will be meaningful for the client, perhaps using symbols as recommended earlier (a monster, an emergency exit sign, a heart, and a surfer, or perhaps a snail coming out of its shell).

Start by asking the child to write or draw thoughts, emotions, and other inner experiences that he usually doesn't like to think or feel, putting each on a separate card. Next, ask him to write or draw important people and activities, again putting each on a separate card. Then ask him to write or draw things he does to fight or struggle with the "yucky inner stuff," one per card. Finally, ask him to write or draw things that allow him to be closer to the important people and activities he wrote or drew on the second set of cards.

Ask him to shuffle the cards, then sort them into the boxes. You can invite parents to join in this part of the game if you like. Consider giving the child the boxes to take home, along with some blank index cards. Then he can continue generating new cards and sorting stuff into the boxes, either on his own or with his parents.

Masks

For this game, you'll need some materials with which the child can create a mask. (For example, you could have blank paper masks and art supplies on hand.) Invite the child to make a mask for his most "yucky" inner obstacle, then use the mask in a role-play. Begin by asking him to put on the mask and behave as the mask's character (the obstacle) would, including tone of voice, what he says, how he walks, his posture, and even how he breathes. In other words, he's embodying the obstacle. For example, if he created an anger mask, he might represent his anger by walking fast, scowling, and speaking very loudly. Listen carefully to what he says so you can use similar language later, when you take on the character of the mask. To draw out the ramifications of acting under the influence of that obstacle, you can invite the child to role-play the behaviors that fit this character; in our example, anger moves might include fighting, screaming, and breaking things (figuratively, of course!).

Next, ask the child what the person he wants to be would do in situations where that mask is likely to put in an appearance. Continuing with the example of anger, the child might say that he'd like to tell his mother how difficult it is for him to do home-work when he's tired.

Next, ask him to take off the mask and give it to you. Put it on yourself, then ask the child to imagine that he's in a situation where he can do what the person he'd like to be would do. Have him role-play his actions as you act out the character depicted by the mask in the same way the child did. As he attempts to move to the right side of his matrix, speak to him using the same tone of voice and saying the same kinds of things. Ask him to do what the person he would like to be would do, including what he would tell the mask. Continuing with our example, the client might then speak to his mother from his heart and tell the mask, "My mother is more important than you right now, and I can choose what to do." Reinforce any success the child has in engaging in toward moves in the role-play, and encourage him to notice when the mask is present in his day-to-day life.

For children who respond well to this game, you can continue to use it in future sessions, having them generate new masks as needed to reflect current inner obstacles.

Concluding Thoughts

Thanks to its versatility, the matrix is an effective tool for working with parents and children. It can help motivate parents to engage in toward moves in the service of their child's best interests, including following the well-established principles of effective parenting set forth in this chapter. And because the matrix is a visual approach, it's well suited to working with children and teenagers, as it can sidestep some of the limitations of verbal language. It can easily be adapted to work with teenagers and younger children, and its flexibility allows it to serve as a springboard for a host of creative exercises that invite children to sort their experience and behaviors in ways that can help them get unstuck and move toward a valued and vital life.

CHAPTER 9

Matrix Work with Couples

We have found the matrix to be ideally suited to couples work. It can speed up the work and get both partners to quickly share a point of view, speak the same language, and develop the ability to discuss their conflicts and challenges in a more distanced way. At the same time, sharing their matrices allows partners to reveal some of their vulnerabilities in a relatively safe way. In this chapter, we describe how we generally use the matrix with couples.

Connecting with Both Partners

When using the matrix with couples, you can start just as you would in individual work, by inviting both partners to describe, in turn, what brings them to therapy. As in individual work, the aim is for you to get a feel for each partner's experience of whatever has brought them to therapy, which you can confirm by reflecting back what they've said and asking whether you've got each partner's perspective right.

Sometimes couples are so stuck that it may be difficult for one or both of them to simply hear the other's point of view without interrupting and arguing. In such cases, you can let them contend with each other for a bit before pausing the exchange and asking whether what's happening in that moment is representative of some of their difficulties. Often couples recognize that it is. If so, that behavior is what we described in chapter 7 as clinically relevant behavior, and it provides a precious opportunity to help both partners shape more workable behaviors in the moment, in session. As a first step, ask them to let each other speak uninterrupted and to give you a chance to reflect what you heard each say.

Once both partners have agreed that you have a good sense of what brings them to you, you can begin to introduce the matrix. But first, and as usual, ask for permission to present the point of view, as described in chapter 1.

Presenting the Matrix

When working with couples, introduce the matrix to both partners. Give each a sheet of paper for detailing their individual matrix. You'll create a third matrix, either on paper or on a whiteboard, on which you'll write down the elements common to both partners' matrices. The following dialogue with Carl and Pam illustrates this approach.

Therapist: This is an active point of view. We call it the matrix. I'll need your participation to set it up. I'm going to invite each of you to draw two intersecting lines like so [draws a bare matrix] on your piece of paper, with arrowheads at the ends of the horizontal line. Above the right arrow, please write "toward," and above the left one write "away." Above the vertical line, write "Five-Senses Experience," and below it write "Inner Experience." Okay?

Pam: Okay.

Carl: Got it.

Therapist: Okay. So as we proceed, you'll each work on your own matrix, and I'll prepare one for what the two of you notice you have in common. Now I'd like each of you to tell me, in no particular order, who or what is important to you. Write your own answers on your matrix. If what your partner says applies to you, let me know, perhaps by saying, "Me too," so I can write it down on the shared point of view I'm recording. Oh, and just to be clear, when I say, "in no particular order," I mean the order in which you mention various things doesn't matter. This isn't a priority list.

Carl: Well, my family and my children are important to me.

Pam: Me too!

Therapist: Great. So, in the lower right quadrant each of you can write, "My family" and "My children," and I'll write those down here too.

Carl: Playing sports with my friends.

Pam: Not to me.

Therapist: Okay. In cases like this, only one of you will write it on your point of view, and I won't write it because it's not important to both of you. Anyone and anything else?

Pam: Our relationship is important to me.

Carl: And to me too!

Therapist: Great, let's all write it down.

You may wonder why the therapist emphasizes that they aren't listing who or what is important in any particular order. In the absence of this clear statement, couples may start arguing about who or what was named first or second, and so on.

After recording who or what is important, move to inner obstacles, in the lower left quadrant, and fill it out in the same way. Here too it's important to establish ground rules and tell both partners that only each of them, individually, can notice what shows up down there, even if what shows up is thoughts about what shows up for their partner. As a general rule, be clear that this point of view is for each partner to notice and show the other, and in no way a tool for engaging in mind reading or projecting onto the other person.

When it comes to writing down away moves and toward moves, be sure to invite both partners to identify their toward and away moves in their relationship. Figure 13 provides an example of a couple's matrix as filled in by their therapist, complete with toward and away moves both partners engage in.

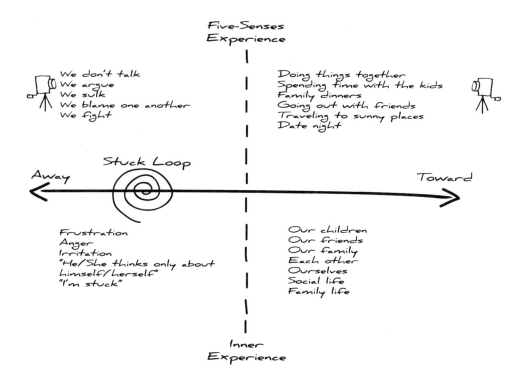

Figure 13.

Seeing their common purpose—who or what is important to both of them—on the joint matrix that you're filling in can help couples commit to therapy and recommit to their relationship. If the lower right quadrant of the joint matrix has few or no entries, ask each person whether it's important that the other be able to pursue separate interests. If both answer yes, you can write that in the lower right quadrant.

Of course, for some couples the lower right quadrant may remain empty, indicating that they have no values in common, in which case therapy may be more about parting amicably, as there would be no good grounds to stay together. Most often, however, they

Matrix Work with Couples   211

have at least a few items in common in the lower right quadrant, allowing them to reconnect with their shared purpose as a couple. And after seeing their own individual experience and their partner's through the lens of the matrix—especially their partner's obstacles and away moves—they typically feel more empathy toward one another. You may feel them relax a bit as they come to realize they're both stuck. As a result, both may get less hooked by the thought that the problem stems entirely from their partner's behavior.

As for seeing each other's toward moves, this is helpful in that it increases the probability that they'll reinforce these behaviors. And seeing their joint toward moves gives them concrete behaviors to engage in that are likely to rapidly improve their relationship.

This is a pretty good time to assign the first home practice exercise, which can simply be noticing their toward and away moves both in their relationship and more broadly. Be sure to mention that, although noticing the other person's toward and away moves is useful, it's rarely effective to point out the other person's away moves, and this can, in fact, lead to getting stuck in renewed conflict. Then describe the alternative: praising and encouraging the other person's toward moves to help increase intimacy and the frequency of those moves.

Identifying Stuck Loops for Two

When one partner engages in an away move in the relationship, it's quite likely that the other will respond with an away move in turn. For example, if one partner feels blamed and withdraws, the other may respond with increased blame, perhaps as a move away from feeling unheard. Clearly, this is likely to trigger another away move by the first person. This kind of dynamic tends to quickly get couples trapped in a painful stuck loop for two. The following dialogue with Pam and Carl illustrates how you can use the matrix to identify these kinds of stuck loops.

Pam:	So, it was another awful weekend. He went off to his motocross with his friends and left me at home to look after the children and do the housework. He just doesn't care. I'm fed up! I don't think I can take much more of this.
Carl:	There she goes again! The whole week I've helped and spent time at home. But all she does is complain.
Pam:	You just don't care about me or your kids, that's what your problem is!
Carl:	And you're just a nag!
Therapist:	Sorry to interrupt, but could you be slipping into one of your stuck loops?
Pam:	What do you mean?

Therapist:	It sounds to me as though the two of you are getting into a familiar place where you're both getting stuck. Would it be fair to say that both of you are feeling stuck right now?
Pam:	I know I am.
Carl:	Yeah, me too.
Therapist:	Okay, good. Would you be willing to sort what's going on with the matrix? *(Both agree.)* So who wants to start?
Pam:	I'll start. Saturday morning he went out with his motocross bike with his friends and only came back after dark, leaving me alone with the kids all day.
Therapist:	It sounds like you had a tough time. So what did you see with your five senses?
Pam:	I saw him leave—not being there!
Therapist:	Okay. And what showed up for you?
Pam:	Feeling abandoned and angry… Feeling like he just doesn't care and that it will never change.
Therapist:	Wow! A lot of stuff showed up. And where does that go in the matrix?
Pam:	*(Points at the lower left quadrant.)* There.
Therapist:	That sounds painful. And what did you do?
Pam:	I told him before he left.
Therapist:	You told him what?
Pam:	That I'm fed up! That I've had enough of this!
Therapist:	And where do you place saying you're fed up?
Pam:	*(Points at the upper left quadrant.)* Up there.
Therapist:	Okay, great. Now let's turn to you, Carl. What showed up for you when Pam did this away move of saying she's fed up?
Carl:	I felt bad. I was fed up too! Look, I spent every weeknight at home and played with the kids. What more does she want?
Therapist:	So where do you place all of that?
Carl:	Bottom left.

Matrix Work with Couples

Therapist:	Okay, great. And what did you do next?
Carl:	I told her to stop nagging.
Therapist:	Okay, and where does that go?
Carl:	Up there on the left.
Therapist:	Excellent. And Pam, what showed up for you when Carl did the away move of saying that? And where does that go?
Pam:	More anger. It goes down there on the left.
Therapist:	And what did you do next, and where does that go?
Pam:	I told him to go away, since he doesn't care about his family. I guess that was an away move too, right?
Therapist:	Okay. And now we could turn to Carl and ask whether he responded to that with more of an away move or a toward move. Carl?
Carl:	(*Chuckles.*) Away! Literally. I left without another word!
Therapist:	It sounds like the two of you got into a stuck loop for two. When certain kinds of painful stuff shows up in our relationships, it's natural to respond to our partner with an away move. In many cases, that away move will make some difficult stuff show up for our partner, who's likely to respond with an away move. And soon enough, we're in a stuck loop for two. That's just natural. And when we're in stuck loops for two, we mainly experience stuckness. Both people engage in away moves, and the entire relationship gets stuck. As long as we remain stuck in away moves, it's impossible to know if the relationship can work. We can only know that away moves get us stuck—no new knowledge gained there. To find out if the relationship can work, toward moves are needed. Only by engaging in toward moves can you see if your partner will respond in kind. If your partner responds to your toward moves with toward moves—maybe not immediately, maybe not always, but a good portion of the time—you can find out whether the relationship can work. It's the only way to know. So noticing your away and toward moves is the first step. Does this make sense?
Pam:	Yes.
Carl:	Yeah, it does.

What happened at the beginning of this exchange is quite common in couples work. Couples tend to get into their stuck loops in session, providing an ideal opportunity to work with the dynamic directly—in the moment in the context of therapy. You can then help them practice identifying what happened and sorting it onto the matrix, and also sow the seeds for the alternative: engaging in toward moves and experiencing new learning about the relationship and whether it can work.

Starting to Get Unstuck

The next step is to introduce positive reinforcement and punishment (though in most cases you may be better off staying away from those terms). As you'll see in the following dialogue, the therapist outlines the benefits of rewarding more workable behavior and the downsides of punishing behaviors that are hurtful. This is often an important part of couples work, as few people understand the power of providing positive reinforcement in creating more workable relationships. Exacerbating this is the human tendency for our attention to be drawn toward problems and stuff to move away from. In couples, this shows up as noticing the other person's away moves, commenting on them, and, usually, criticizing them. Of course, if that worked, there would be little need for couples therapy. However, as that need does exist in unfortunate abundance, we'll return to Pam and Carl's therapy session.

Therapist:	Okay, good. So now let's turn to toward moves you each noticed yourself or your partner doing over the past week. Who wants to start?
Pam:	I will. I noticed Carl played with the kids more.
Carl:	Yes, I did! I'm glad you noticed it.
Therapist:	Great! And was this a toward move for you, Carl?
Carl:	Yes, of course, and I enjoyed it.
Therapist:	Excellent. So Pam, what showed up for you when you saw Carl do that?
Pam:	I was happy. But I also thought, "Why doesn't he do this more often?"
Therapist:	Okay, so where would you place that?
Pam:	I guess happy goes over there on the right.
Therapist:	And the thought "Why doesn't he do this more often?" Where does that go?
Pam:	Bottom left.
Therapist:	Cool. And what did you do next?
Pam:	Nothing.
Therapist:	Did you say anything?

Pam:	No.
Therapist:	But you felt happy, right? Here's another question. Would you like Carl to do more of those toward moves?
Pam:	For sure.
Therapist:	How about you, Carl? Did you notice any toward moves of Pam's?
Carl:	When I called to say I was overwhelmed at work one day, Pam suggested that I stay later, even though she was relying on me to be home early that night, and I knew it.
Therapist:	How did that feel to you?
Carl:	Good. It was a huge relief.
Therapist:	And what did you do or say?
Carl:	Nothing much.
Therapist:	Okay. Let me ask both of you this then: When you do these kinds of toward moves, would you rather your partner noticed them and showed appreciation for them, or would you rather the other person carried on as if nothing had happened?
Pam:	A little appreciation would be nice.
Carl:	Agreed.
Therapist:	And regarding away moves, would you rather your partner comment on them or say nothing?
Pam:	If we comment on them, we're more likely to get into an argument.
Carl:	Right.
Therapist:	So really noticing and appreciating toward moves can make those more likely and help us get into a toward loop for two, whereas focusing on away moves and criticizing them is more likely to get us into a stuck loop for two. That's kind of strange, because most of us tend to pay more attention to our partner's away moves and comment most heavily on those. Would you say that's the case for you two?
Pam:	Hmm... Yes. It's true that complaining about what the other person is doing tends to land us in a lot of arguments.
Therapist:	Well, you don't have to believe me about this. Just do an experiment. In one part of the experiment both of you would focus on appreciating the

other person's toward moves for a while and just let each other's away moves be. In the second part of the experiment, you would ignore each other's toward moves and comment solely on the away moves. Which of those do you want to start with for the coming week?

Carl: I guess we tried the second option already. Maybe try supporting the toward moves and shutting up about the rest?

Therapist: Excellent. I'm looking forward to hearing what you notice.

Hooks and Couples

With couples, hooks can be presented in essentially the same way as in chapter 3. However, it's important to clarify that hooks are something for each partner to notice individually. Few couples have found it useful to tease out each other's hooks or to say the other person must be hooked. Although hooks may come in the form of five-senses experience, we can only notice them—and whether we bite them—as individuals, because only individuals can tell if their behavior is what they would have done if they hadn't gotten hooked.

With that in mind, working with hooks, filling in the Hooks Worksheet, and sharing their hooks with one another can help both partners develop greater empathy for each other. The key is that this work be done as a means of self-discovery, not as a means of proving either partner wrong or right.

Verbal Aikido for Couples

Getting both partners to notice their inner experience, their own behavior, and their partner's behavior is an important part of couples work. Verbal aikido for two is ideally suited for this. It has the added advantage of helping both partners identify and describe, in front of each other, what behavior they'd engage in if they didn't get hooked. It's also a way to promote perspective taking and empathy, as you'll see in the following dialogue.

In this example, we turn to Joan and Herb. As a couple, one of the places they get stuck is around how they negotiate Herb's return from the office. He has a high-pressure job and regularly gets home after Joan, who's a shop manager working fixed hours. After their therapist shares the worksheet and briefly outlines the basic aikido moves, she invites Joan and Herb to choose a specific situation to practice on. Note that throughout the exchange, the therapist is pointing at the questions on the Verbal Aikido Worksheet.

Therapist: Okay, so what situation would you like to look at with these basic moves?

Joan: Let's look at what happens when Herb comes home.

Herb:	Okay.
Therapist:	Who wants to do the first round and respond to these questions?
Joan:	I'll start.
Therapist:	Okay, so when did this situation last come up? Where were you?
Joan:	Yesterday. I was in the kitchen.
Therapist:	Good. What time was it?
Joan:	About seven o'clock.
Therapist:	Okay, and what could you notice with your five senses?
Joan:	I heard Herb open the door, come up the stairs, say hi from a distance, and disappear into his study.
Therapist:	And did you notice any hooks?
Joan:	Yes, of course! I thought, "He doesn't care about me and isn't even interested in my day."
Therapist:	Okay, and how did those hooks feel?
Joan:	I felt angry.
Therapist:	And where was that in your body?
Joan:	*(Points to the top of her stomach.)* Here.
Therapist:	Great, and did you bite the hooks yesterday?
Joan:	Yes.
Therapist:	What did you do next?
Joan:	I started sulking.
Therapist:	What did that look like on the video camera?
Joan:	When he came out of his study and asked me about my day, I looked down and didn't say anything.
Therapist:	And what would the person you want to be have done?
Joan:	I would have asked about his day and told him about mine.
Therapist:	What's important to you in being able to do that?
Joan:	Having a smooth relationship, sharing, and not fighting.

Therapist:	How does it feel to you to say that this is important to you?
Joan:	It feels warm here (*pointing to her heart*).
Therapist:	Excellent. One last question: How was it for you to practice these verbal aikido moves?
Joan:	Not too bad!
Therapist:	You did a great job. Herb, now it's your turn. Are you still up for it?
Herb:	Sure.
Therapist:	Okay, so what did you notice with your five senses as you came home?
Herb:	I guess I saw the door and the stairs. I heard Joan in the kitchen.
Therapist:	Did any hooks show up?
Herb:	Well, when I get home, I have my routine. I hang my coat and take my shoes off. Then I go put my wallet in my study and look at my mail, which Joan puts on my desk for me.
Joan:	Yes, he's almost OCD about this!
Herb:	I just like to do this in a certain order.
Therapist:	Can any of these be hooks for you?
Herb:	I guess they could be. I'm the organized one.
Therapist:	Okay. So what do you do when you bite those hooks?
Herb:	I just go into my study and do my stuff.
Therapist:	Excellent. And what would the person you want to be do?
Herb:	Well, seeing how hard this is for Joan, I guess I could say hello first. I could give her a kiss and tell her that I'll be back shortly to ask her about her day.
Therapist:	Who or what's important to you in being able to do that?
Herb:	Who's important is Joan. What's important is to let her know that she's important to me and that I appreciate her and everything she does.
Therapist:	How does it feel to say that this is important to you?
Herb:	It feels warm here (*pointing to his heart*).

Therapist:	Excellent. So, Herb, how was it for you to practice these verbal aikido moves?
Herb:	It was okay.

Remember that verbal aikido need not be practiced on the most difficult situations. It's just as effective at training noticing when used for everyday sticky situations as it is when used for more challenging material. In fact, at first it may be easier to practice on a lower-intensity situation, especially when couples are highly stuck. However, do bear in mind that it's usually best to let the couple choose the situation they want to work on. (In the next section we'll give an example of how the matrix can be used to help discuss thorny issues in a more defused and empathetic way.)

Using verbal aikido allows both partners to reveal what's difficult for them and what's important. It also allows both to describe what an improved behavior would look like so that they can then notice their partner doing this and reinforce it. The home practice would be for both partners to use the verbal aikido moves in sticky situations. If they communicate well at this stage of therapy, they can use the Verbal Aikido for Two Worksheet together to share about sticky situations.

Be sure to communicate that verbal aikido works best if each person practices the basic moves for himself or herself, rather than trying to force particular moves on the other. An effective and humorous way to do this is to suggest that each partner ask the questions only of himself or herself—unless they're paying each other the same amount as they're paying you to ask these questions.

Working Through Challenging Material by Sorting with the Matrix

When people are stuck in a conflict, it's only natural for them to look for allies, and they may turn to you for this kind of support. Beware. The last thing you want to do is to get into a position in which one partner sees you as allied with the other. Be open about that risk and let the couple know you only work in the service of what's important to both of them, not the personal interests of either of them.

Still, when couples are in conflict in session, therapists tend to mediate the exchange by speaking in turn for each partner until both feel heard and validated. Using the matrix to sort difficult material can be especially effective in such situations. Whereas the tendency might otherwise be for both partners to immediately slip into one of their stuck loops for two, they can instead quickly share their experience around hot-button issues while sidestepping previous patterns. Your role as a therapist is thus to orient the couple toward sorting on the matrix, rather than reformulating what each person says in such a way that both can be heard and feel validated.

We'll illustrate this approach using a dialogue with Jean and Clark, who are struggling in the wake of Clark's infidelity. As you'll see, this dialogue also illustrates a point we emphasized earlier: that couples often engage in habitual stuck loops in session, providing an excellent opportunity to intervene in those patterns of unworkable behavior.

Jean:	I don't know if I can ever forgive you for cheating on me.
Clark:	You keep bringing this up. How long am I going to have to pay for it?
Jean:	You act as though it was nothing!
Clark:	You keep hammering on about it. I've said I was sorry many times, but it seems like it will never be enough.
Jean:	You have no idea how deeply hurt I feel.
Clark:	What more can I say? You always come back to this.
Therapist:	Can I interrupt for a second? Is it possible that the exchange you're having right now is similar to exchanges you have in your everyday life whenever this subject shows up?
Clark:	Absolutely!
Therapist:	And so you both get stuck in this way, right? That sounds painful.
Jean:	I'm not sure what to do. I feel like he wants to pretend it never happened.
Clark:	I feel like she wants me to carry this around my neck forever!
Therapist:	Okay. Would you both be willing to sort this on the matrix?
Jean:	Sure.
Clark:	Okay.
Therapist:	So which of you wants to start with what you have to say about this?
Clark:	I will. I feel like Jean will never forgive me and that she'll bring it up at every opportunity.

Because Clark said something that's likely to get Jean hooked, the therapist turns to Jean and guides her in practicing the basic verbal aikido moves, which are a way of sorting onto the matrix.

Therapist:	Okay. Jean, what shows up for you when you hear Clark say those words?
Jean:	I feel like he's pretending nothing happened.
Therapist:	Is that a hook for you?

Jean:	A very big hook! And not just a hook—it happened, after all.
Therapist:	Good. And how does that feel? Where is it in your body?
Jean:	I feel angry, sad, and scared. It's here *(pointing)* in my throat and in my heart. *(Starts tearing up.)*
Therapist:	Okay, and what do you do next when you get hooked?
Jean:	I tell him that he doesn't care and I can't trust him.
Therapist:	Okay. And what would the partner you want to be do or say?
Jean:	*(Pauses.)* She would say, "I want to forgive him and trust him again, but I was badly hurt and I still hurt."
Therapist:	What's important to you about saying that?
Jean:	Being authentic. Being understood.
Therapist:	How does that feel, and where is it in your body?
Jean:	It's here and here *(crying and pointing to her stomach and heart)*.
Therapist:	Okay. So would you be willing to tell Clark what the person you want to be would say? If yes, just go ahead and tell him.
Jean:	Clark, I want to forgive you, but I need you to see how hurt I am still and how hard it is.
Therapist:	Okay. Now Clark, how do you respond to Jean's toward move?
Clark:	Honey, I'm sorry that you feel so bad. I know how hard this has been for you. There isn't one moment that I don't feel guilty about what I did. I can't believe you could ever want to forgive me.
Jean:	I know it's hard for you too. I love you, and I love the family and the life we've made together. I know we can survive this.
Therapist:	So, did you both just engage in toward moves or away moves?
Jean:	Toward!
Clark:	Yes, toward.
Therapist:	Excellent. Clark, what hooks did you notice?
Clark:	Guilt. Shame. Feeling like I can never forgive myself.
Therapist:	How did that feel, and where is it in your body?

Clark: It feels awful. It's here *(pointing to his throat)*.

Therapist: And if you had bitten those hooks, what would you have said?

Clark: The usual stuff, I guess: "Why don't you give me a break? I've apologized already. Will you ever stop blaming me?" The point is, I already blame myself so much…

Therapist: Let's pause here for a second. It seems like, this time, both of you found a way to engage in toward moves when this painful subject showed up. Do you feel it brought you closer together or pushed you farther away from one another?

Jean: Closer.

Clark: Yes, I agree.

Therapist: Excellent. I wonder how it was for each of you to hear about your partner's hooks. Clark?

Clark: It was hard, but it made me realize how much she's still hurting.

Therapist: Jean?

Jean: I could see that he also feels really bad about it.

Therapist: So next time this shows up, do you think you can do a bit of what you just did here with me today?

Jean: I'll try.

Clark: I will too.

In this exchange, Clark and Jean got stuck because they didn't validate each other. Of course, the validation needed here is for each partner to reflect what the other one feels, not to seek a way to rationalize or excuse what happened. Once Clark and Jean could do this, they were able to move toward one another. In some cases, one or both partners won't know how to validate. If so, you can prompt validation by suggesting that both simply repeat what the other said, with special emphasis on the emotions their partner expressed. Then, after repeating this back, they can check in and see how their partner felt upon hearing those thoughts and feelings reflected back. Did the reflection feel fairly accurate? If not, have them repeat the process until they both feel validated. At times you'll need to provide validation yourself and check to see whether what you reflected is indeed validating. Then invite the partner who's practicing validation to repeat something close to your words and check whether that worked to make the other partner feel validated. Also suggest that they practice validation between sessions.

CHAPTER 10

The Matrix in Life Coaching

This chapter outlines a session-by-session format for using the matrix in life coaching, followed by two extended examples to help demonstrate the approach. When using ACT in coaching work, we refer to acceptance and commitment training, rather than acceptance and commitment therapy. The difference reflects the target of the behavioral intervention. Therapists often seek to treat behavioral disorders that are significantly impairing clients' functioning. Coaching is targeted at enhancing behaviors in people who are functioning well and seeking to up their game. The matrix is perfect for helping people quickly see the big picture—including gaining some deep knowledge about where they want to go in their life and career, along with the internal and external barriers they face—and then deriving new behaviors that move them forward.

When using the matrix for coaching, the first task is to form a flexible alliance with clients. By "flexible," we mean the relationship will serve to help clients find new behaviors that work. Such work inherently requires both flexibility and openness. Rather than intellectually explaining this flexibility and openness, we simply work the matrix, cultivating openness and flexibility as a natural part of the process.

Session 1: Coaching Goals

Since coaching is very goal oriented, the usual matrix approach of starting in the lower right quadrant is ideally suited to the work. After presenting the matrix diagram, we ask, "Who is important to you?" After a few minutes of discussing who's important, we then ask, "How do your career and life aspirations line up with who's important?" Rather than treating all of this (values and values-consistent behavior) as a static situation, we stress that it can change over time, as the client learns and discovers. After setting the context in this way, we often refer to the work as being about a chosen life purpose. While it might more accurately be called "the purpose that you're choosing over time," we find that clients quickly grasp that "chosen life purpose" is a flexible term.

At this point, you can share a bit about who's important to you, your aspirations, and how you've noticed that these change over time. Since this is a coaching environment, clients will have some curiosity about how you've gone about being successful. In coaching, self-disclosure can help show clients that you use the same coaching process with yourself.

Next, we address the lower left quadrant with the question "What shows up inside you and gets in the way?" Garden-variety fear always shows up, but fear of failure, rejection, or even success can also show up. Impatience, anger, and envy are other common answers. Again, share a bit about yourself during this conversation, including that new barriers crop up for you often, but you address them with the very process you're showing the client now.

Next, move to the upper left quadrant, explaining that it contains behaviors done to decrease any unwanted feelings identified in the lower left, emphasizing that these are observable behaviors. At this point, we recommend introducing the concept of time spent on unnecessary away moves. Point out that many away moves are workable, such as avoiding oncoming cars, not running with scissors, and other life-saving behaviors, but that we all also avoid anxiety when it would be more workable to accept it and choose to move toward what's important. Tell clients that there's no need to keep track of the time lost to unnecessary away moves, because awareness of this lost time will happen automatically over time as they work the matrix.

Finally, discuss the upper right quadrant, explaining that it contains behaviors that could be done to move toward who or what is important. Start with simple behaviors like walking and talking. Later you can work with clients to add more complex behaviors that can help them move toward chosen life purposes.

The Vertical and Horizontal Lines

While you need not talk about the function of the lines of the matrix during coaching work, you certainly can if it enhances the work for you. Regarding the vertical line, noticing the difference between five-senses and inner experiences can help clients stay grounded in the present moment. And noticing the difference between how it feels to move away and how it feels to move toward helps them be aware of what's motivating them from moment to moment. In particular, you may want to point out that toward moves have an element of satisfaction, whereas away moves have an element of relief. Those who have studied psychology will recognize that the right side involves positive reinforcement, while the left is largely about negative reinforcement.

Whether or not you choose to review the vertical and horizontal lines, do touch upon all four quadrants, with particular emphasis on the lower right quadrant. At this point, some clients may not have a clearly defined life purpose. That's fine. The general idea of purpose provides a target criterion to begin with. New behaviors can be tried and tested to see if they work for creating a sense of purpose. Then these clients can begin to more clearly define their life purpose.

In any discussion of purpose, help clients see the importance of holding any given purpose lightly and flexibly. Of course, life purposes need to be clear and kept in mind.

Yet holding them tightly may stand in the way of flexibility. After all, life circumstances can sometimes change quickly, and in such situations flexibility is key.

Homework

Holding things lightly extends to homework. (It also extends to terminology—for example, choosing to use the term "homework" with coaching clients because, for these clients, it's less likely to lead to resistance.) As established in earlier chapters, matrix practitioners fully realize and expect that sometimes homework isn't done. Since at its core ACT is a learning model, we are simply noticing what is being learned. Thus, one can notice and learn as homework is completed or not completed. You can even tell clients that they either will or will not do homework and that either is workable because learning will occur in both cases. So instead of following a rigid "homework must be done" rule, we suggest the more flexible principle that learning occurs all the time, and clients' job is to notice.

As a first exercise, we recommend inviting coaching clients to notice who or what is important to them between the first and second session. You may notice that this is different than the home practices in part 1 of the book, which had a focus on noticing toward and away moves. In coaching, the focus is on direction. Any life purpose must take who or what is important into account, so this homework will help clients identify and define their life purpose.

Session 2: Hooks

In session 2, we review life purpose, introduce hooks, and look at how content in the lower left quadrant can come to control behavior. This session also provides opportunities to practice flexibility and yessing when coaching clients.

Reviewing the Homework

As mentioned above, in matrix-oriented coaching you'll accept that homework is either done or not done. So simply ask, "What did you notice while doing or not doing the homework?" This question prompts clients to look back at the past few days and bring to mind the homework.

If clients forgot the homework entirely, you can introduce hooks and review some that are common. Most clients will recall having encountered hooks over the past week. Maybe some showed up and got in the way of doing the homework. Often clients won't have noticed hooks or that they bit them. Tell them that's okay, that noticing hooks in the moment is a skill that takes some practice to develop. For clients who are able to identify some hooks, look at a couple that they noticed, asking them to recall first their five-senses experience when encountering the hook, and then their inner experience. Then ask them to recall what behavior they engaged in right after the hook showed up. After this, share that they're now more likely to notice hooks in the moment, especially if they're aware of their most common hooks and when those are most likely to show up.

We review homework this way because the goal is to start noticing hooks and getting hooked in the moment, and that takes practice. More broadly, hooks can serve as a ready reminder for noticing the process of responding in context.

Reviewing Life Purpose

After debriefing the homework—and presenting hooks if the debriefing opened the door to that—revisit life purpose. After offering a reminder that life purpose is an ongoing process, ask clients if they're ready to narrow down to the specific purpose they want to focus on in coaching. If they aren't ready yet, make it clear that this is okay.

Looking at Hooks

The primary focus of session 2 is the lower left quadrant: what shows up and gets in the way. Start by reviewing whatever clients identified in session 1. If you didn't introduce hooks in the homework review, do so now. Then you can move to helping clients get a better feel for their obstacles to success, satisfaction, and even happiness. You can ask if any of their inner obstacles are showing up as hooks. If they don't experience their internal obstacles as hooks, then how are those obstacles showing up and interfering with moving toward their purpose? To zero in on this, you can ask clients to recall a typical time of day when the obstacle shows up, a typical place where it shows up in the world, and a typical area where they feel it in their body.

Obstacles, especially internal ones, are sneaky and can easily go unnoticed. When you ask clients to recall both external and internal details of their obstacles, you help them become more apt at noticing their obstacles when they show up.

At this point, you can start addressing behaviors in response to obstacles. Inquire about them, then map them to the upper left quadrant. Reiterate that this is about observable behaviors—things clients could be seen doing on a video camera—not internal struggles with their barriers. In session 2, clients may not yet be aware of a lot of their away behaviors, and that's fine. In this case your work is about setting the stage for them to notice these behaviors in the future.

You might give yourself as an example and share about your own away behaviors in response to a variety of obstacles that show up inside you. This will help clients see that attempting to avoid obstacles is human nature and something everyone does, including you. The main thing is to start noticing both obstacles and avoidance. Throughout, keep returning to workability. The point of session 2 is to get clients to notice how their away behaviors work in the overall process of moving toward their life purpose. Some of these behaviors will work and some won't. In many cases, it depends on the situation. For example, sometimes it works to avoid a bully, and other times it works to confront the bully. Carefully noticing their away moves will help clients learn what works.

Moving Toward Purpose

At this point, you might review what clients could do to move toward their purpose—observable behaviors in the upper right of the matrix. If clients haven't already started deriving new behaviors and telling you about them, return to the basics and help them practice simply noticing the difference between five-senses and mental experience and the difference in how it feels to move away and how it feels to move toward. Why return to the basics? You may have noticed that you yourself experience more satisfaction when engaged in behaviors that you came up with on your own, as opposed to following someone else's suggestions. So stick with the basics until clients spontaneously provide content in the upper right quadrant, and go with whatever they come up with.

That said, the matrix generally promotes rapid increases in psychological flexibility. Therefore, by the end of session 2, clients are likely to be coming up with new behaviors to try.

Homework

We recommend asking clients to notice their hooks and what they do next as homework. You can offer the Hooks Worksheet from chapter 3, if you like. Noticing hooks is probably the easiest way for people to practice noticing in the moment and gain some distance from their thoughts. At this point, clients will be somewhat familiar with the main discriminations, so ask them to consider workability as well. You can do this by saying something like "When you're noticing the hook, you might notice your five-senses experience and any urge to move away or toward. Then notice your next behavior. Ultimately, you may start noticing whether those behaviors are helping you move toward your life purpose."

Session 3: Getting on Track

The most important part of almost anything we do in life is staying on track. First we need to get on track, and then we go about the business of staying on track. Although life doesn't provide us with the rigid rails that keep a train on course, we can use the matrix to stay close to the path we've chosen by noticing the consequences of what we do in the moment. In other words, when clients get off track, the matrix perspective can help them quickly notice the consequences and correct their course.

Reviewing the Homework

Begin with a quick review of the homework. For this debrief, ask clients to sort what they noticed about hooks onto the matrix. This could be simply sorting their five-senses versus mental experiencing and away versus toward behavior when the hook shows up and also afterward. This simple level of sorting will work well. However, you can also have them sort who or what is important, what shows up inside and gets in the way, away moves, and toward moves. Whether the sorting is simple or more complex, it's likely to foster greater psychological flexibility, allowing clients to think up potential new toward behaviors. At this point, it's important for neither the client nor the coach to prejudge the workability of these new behaviors. No one can know for sure whether new behaviors will work in a given context. So simply invite clients to experiment with these new behaviors and notice their workability.

Looking at Consequences

The preceding homework debrief opens the door to a discussion of how consequences are the best way to learn behaviors that work. As you enter this discussion, be sure to point out some of the potential traps. For example, we humans tend to believe what our minds tell us about consequences, rather than really noticing consequences with our five senses. Said in a less polite way, we tend to bullshit ourselves. We can convince ourselves that a little success is a lot. Worse, we can find ways to see unworkable as workable and then keep doing what doesn't work. The simple way out of these traps is to pay attention to what we notice with our five senses after trying a new behavior. By doing so, we obtain more information and can more quickly learn what works.

As you can see, learning by paying attention to the consequences of behavior is strikingly different from traditional coaching. Traditional approaches typically involve carefully setting up a plan and then motivating clients to stick with the plan. In contrast, the matrix approach involves roughing out a plan, increasing psychological flexibility, letting new behaviors percolate, and then testing them by noticing their consequences with five-senses and inner experiencing. As a matrix coach, you aren't the source of motivation; rather, you help clients find intrinsic motivation. In the short term, they immediately move toward who or what is important to them. In the long term, they move toward their chosen life purpose—an idea of what a valued life would look like in the future.

Using Sorting to Promote Tracking

Sorting can promote tracking, so this is also a focus in session 3. Sorting will occur naturally as you increasingly direct clients toward the categories of the matrix: who or what is important, what shows up and gets in the way, away behaviors, and toward behaviors. Everything we humans experience and do can be sorted into these categories. And because humans love to sort and put puzzles together, looking at our experience through the lens of the matrix comes fairly easily. Further, there's a sense of satisfaction in getting stuff into the "right" areas of the matrix.

That said, throughout this work do keep in mind there's no "correct" way for clients to sort. In a way, even the terms used to describe the categories and the categories themselves aren't important. What matters most is the act of sorting, as it promotes distancing, or defusion. To help clients see this and sidestep any tendency to overly focus on the accuracy of their sorting, you might offer a metaphor about the physical exercise of walking: "It's the overall process of walking that's important, not that steps were put in the right places." Even so, knowing this won't deter your clients (or you) from trying to achieve the correct sort. Noticing that and returning to the knowledge that there really isn't a wrong way to sort can be helpful in increasing flexibility.

As a coach, your job is done once you ask clients to sort an experience. For example, let's say a client tells you, "My husband and I went to dinner last night." You would respond, "That's nice to hear. Just to practice using the matrix a bit, where would you put your husband? And where would you put going to dinner with him last night?" If you see that the client is stumped, you can give a hint, such as "Who's important goes down here." Soon clients will get the hang of sorting. From the moment you ask clients to engage in sorting, they take a different perspective on their experience. Curiosity and psychological flexibility increase, leading to behavioral flexibility.

As always, assign some type of noticing homework, such as noticing hooks and, to promote tracking, noticing consequences. For example, you might ask clients to notice whether hooks show up that take them off track and whether they notice getting back on track after a hook shows up, or you can ask them to notice the consequence of staying hooked a long time. However, at this point in coaching we often let clients come up with the homework. Whatever the homework may be, remind clients that they will learn whether or not they engage in the homework.

Session 4: Overcoming External Barriers

In session 1 we did an overview of the psychological flexibility point of view, then focused on life purpose and goals in terms of who or what is important. In session 2 we reviewed the matrix and focused on hooks and internal barriers. In session 3 we made sure clients can easily engage in sorting, enhancing their ability to notice the consequences of new behavior. In session 4 we review the matrix and then turn to a topic not generally covered in other matrix work: external barriers, which are mapped onto the upper right quadrant. This makes sense in the context of life coaching, where the work is often about helping people move toward concrete goals, rather than identifying and clarifying underlying values.

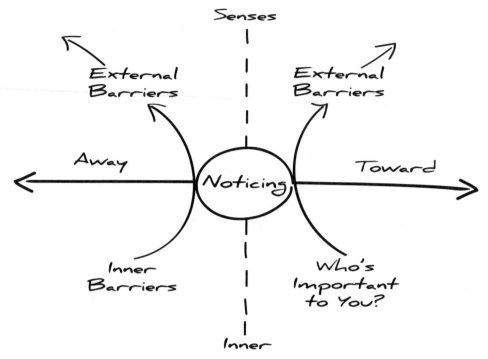

Figure 14.

Bringing in External Barriers

Of course, even in this context, underlying values inform goals, and inner barriers are often more limiting than external barriers. That's why we don't introduce external barriers until the matrix is well established. In addition, humans are expert at finding external barriers and then blaming them for lack of progress. That said, sometimes clients do face genuine external barriers and need help with problem solving to achieve workable toward or away moves, as represented by figure 14. Then again, sometimes simply recognizing an external barrier suffices to increase psychological flexibility to the point where the person can come up with a new behavior to overcome the barrier. And sometimes persistence or a minor change in behavior is all that's needed, in which case the motivation provided by purpose will carry the day.

To help clients overcome an external barrier, it's best to encourage them to use their five senses to focus on it. If they don't, they may end up getting caught up in internal barriers that arise in relation to the external obstacle. We've all done it: we encounter an external obstacle that's easily remedied, like a flat tire, and the mind goes wild with internal barriers like panicky thoughts that lead to feeling doomed and slumping down, rather than fixing the tire. By guiding clients to first carefully notice the external obstacle with their five senses, you put them in a much better position to notice any thoughts and feelings as just part of the picture that need not interfere with solving the problem. This is a way of purposely overcorrecting in order to stay grounded in sensory experience.

Bringing Flexibility to Bear on External Barriers

After defining an external barrier using the five senses, it takes some mental processing to identify and choose a solution from preexisting behaviors or to come up with a new one. Psychological flexibility is key here. As ever, you can help clients develop more psychological flexibility by reminding them to notice the difference between five-senses and mental experiencing, and to notice or recall the difference in how it feels to move toward and how it feels to move away. Practicing these basic matrix discriminations will increase the chances that clients can come up with a broad range of potential solutions.

When one or more solutions have shown up, encourage clients to try them, perhaps offering a gentle reminder to hold potential solutions lightly. A solution needs to be workable, and workability can only be determined through five-senses, real-life experience, along with some mental processing. This can help prevent clients from jumping to conclusions or getting caught in other cognitive traps that can easily show up during problem solving and hook them. If such hooks show up, they can be noticed for what they are. Such noticing helps with workable problem solving.

Additional Sessions: Nurturing the Process

The four sessions we've just outlined engage clients in viewing their life and life purpose from the psychological flexibility point of view. The ultimate purpose is to increase psychological flexibility so that clients can come up with new behaviors and test them for workability. Any work you do after session 4 can then be aimed at providing a nurturing environment so that this process takes hold and becomes second nature.

Nurturing is very important. As Anthony Biglan discusses in *The Nurture Effect* (2015), coercive environments don't foster the discovery of workable new behaviors. In all likelihood, no life coach actively seeks to be coercive; however, coercion can sneak into the coaching process. We need look no further than assigning homework to clients. If doing the homework is required for the work to proceed, an element of coercion sneaks in. Clients may feel punished when they don't do the homework. Another example relates to problem solving, where it's easy to slip into making recommendations. Yet saying things like "You should try doing it this way" may leave clients feeling coerced, in which case they may engage in behaviors to move away from that coercion or under the control of that coercion. It's a fine line to tread, given that people often seek coaching because they want to be told what to do. While some of that can be workable, too much can quickly become unworkable.

People Come First

Life coaching often revolves around some type of business or career goal. This can place matrix coaching in the context of a mechanistic worldview that has dominated most business thinking since the industrial revolution. This orientation is often very workable, and it's a natural outgrowth of the creation of increasingly efficient machines to do so much work. Henry Ford and his ilk focused on the interplay of machines and people to create highly efficient processes for turning out high-quality products and services. The downside is that people easily come to be treated as machines. When that happens, they feel disrespected, they don't feel safe, and they don't feel nurtured. Life coaches can help some by making sure their clients learn the importance of showing respect. People don't learn this by being told about it or reading about it; they need to practice showing respect and notice how others respond to it. This all but guarantees that they'll experience firsthand that putting respect (people) first is very workable.

In his book *Toyota Kata* (2010), Mike Rother notes that the creator of the Toyota process (which is generally termed "lean management" in the West) prescribes beginning by going to the *gemba* and asking questions with respect. *Gemba* simply means "where the work is happening." So this prescription means being respectful of employees who are actually doing the work, which includes asking them about their process. What does this have to do with life coaching? The people you coach will interact with others. One of the best ways to interact with others is to get out of one's head and be with people, without making assumptions and instead asking everyone questions that demonstrate interest and respect. Of course, we're not saying you should coerce clients into doing this. Perhaps all that's needed is a casual mention that tons of research has shown that nurturing others is the road to anyone's success.

Life Coaching Examples

To put the matrix approach to life coaching in context, let's take a look at how you might work with a couple of fictional clients, first John, and then Joy, who are both working on personal as well as career goals.

John

From your intake form you know that John is an accountant. He's come to you because he feels that he isn't moving up the career ladder as he'd envisioned in accounting school. He's been an accountant for ten years and is now thirty-four.

When he arrives for his first session, John is well dressed and groomed. You notice yourself thinking that he looks like an accountant you might see in a movie. As is your usual practice, you ask him if it's okay to show him the point of view that you work from, called the matrix. John readily agrees. You review the basic matrix with him: five-senses experiencing, then mental experiencing, and then noticing the difference. Next, you ask him to recall how it feels to move toward someone who's important to him, and he immediately says, "That's easy: Joy, it's a joy to move toward her." Then you ask him to recall how it feels to move away from some unwanted feeling, like fear. Then you ask him to notice the difference. Next, you ask him who's important to him, and he says "Joy" again.

You: Is Joy your wife?

John: No. She's not even my girlfriend, but she's important.

You: Great! Is anyone else important to you?

John: My mom. My dad died a year ago.

You: I'm sorry to hear that. Anyone else?

John: Well, I have a coworker who's also a friend.

You: This is a great list! We can always add to this list as we work together.

John: I forgot my cat. She's important.

You: You bet. Cats and dogs are family.

John: Now that you say family, my brothers and sister are important.

You: Is anyone or anything else important to you?

John: Yes. My work. That's one of the main reasons I'm here.

You: Okay, we've got all of those written up on the matrix. Now, over here in the lower left we put the stuff like fear—inner experiences that can show up and get in the way of moving toward who's important to you. For example, when you were younger you might have thought about asking someone on a date. Maybe fear showed up, and maybe it got in the way.

John: I have that now. I'd like to ask Joy out, but I haven't gotten around to it. She's the one who gave me your name.

You: Really? That's flattering.

John: Yeah, she did a stress management presentation where I work. I went up to talk to her afterward. She was really nice to me. She ended up giving me your name when I told her I wanted to get ahead at work. She showed us the matrix in her presentation, so I've sort of done this before.

You: Great! I don't recall meeting a Joy. But I'm glad she sent you my way. Can you think of other stuff that shows up inside of you and gets in the way?

John: At work, anxiety and stress get in the way. They slow me down too much. Accounts are supposed to be methodical, but I think my boss thinks I'm too slow.

You:	Great! Any other stuff that shows up and gets in the way?
John:	Tiredness. I get tired in the afternoon, and that slows me down too. Also, thinking that I'm not good enough shows up a lot.
You:	This is a great list of internal stuff that can get in the way. You can always add more later. When we go up here, to the upper part of the matrix, we list the behaviors you do—the stuff everyone can see you doing. So here in the upper left we put your typical away moves—the stuff you do to reduce or get rid of the stuff down here in the lower left. Can you think of behaviors you do to move away?
John:	I avoid a lot to get away from anxiety.
You:	Great! What does your avoidance look like?
John:	At the office, I keep to myself. That way people don't expect so much from me. I guess I keep to myself in general. I stay at home a lot. Sometimes I watch movies… Oh yeah, I also ride my bike to get rid of stress. I got brave and mentioned that during the stress management presentation.
You:	The one Joy did?
John:	Yes!
You:	This is great stuff. Anything else?
John:	Well, I daydream a bit.
You:	Okay, and how does it look when you're daydreaming?
John:	I stare off into the distance, I guess. Do you think others notice?
You:	Maybe, but most of us get wrapped up in our minds and forget to notice others, so maybe not. Now we'll go to the upper right. This is where we write the stuff that you could do to move toward who or what is important to you. First we look at what you wrote in the lower right. Joy, your family, your cat, and your friend at work are important, and so is your work. Those are a good start. What might you do to move toward any of those?
John:	I could ask Joy out on a date. For work, I could focus on going faster by being less of a perfectionist.
You:	So, if you were to set about asking Joy out or working faster, do you think you might notice anything from the lower left showing up and getting in the way of doing those things?

John:	(*Laughs out loud.*) Well, fear has already shown up. That's why I haven't asked her out. I'm afraid she'll say no!
You:	Great noticing! You're already getting the hang of this. What else might show up?
John:	Fear of making a mistake, of not being perfect at work. Going fast scares me.
You:	Cool. You've got some great noticing lined up. Now consider this: Have you ever had something happen that grabbed you emotionally and stuck with you for a while, like getting cut off in traffic or seeing an attractive person walk by? Maybe it stuck with you so much that later you saw a friend and told that person about what happened?
John:	That happens all the time. Other drivers piss me off a lot.
You:	Great! That's just what I'm talking about. We call those hooks. Do you think you'll have the opportunity to notice some hooks over the next week?
John:	You bet!
You:	Would you like to schedule a follow-up session?
John:	Yes.

Thus ends session 1. We're going to skip ahead to session 4. Although you might typically sequence the sessions differently, John had prior experience with the matrix and was getting it well. So in session 2 you went ahead and focused on internal barriers, and in session 3 you focused on external barriers. You also returned to other aspects of the matrix during those sessions to reinforce the point of view. As we've mentioned throughout, the matrix is about being flexible and responding and tracking in the moment—for practitioners and clients alike—so you changed the sequence of your sessions to fit the client's needs and context. Now you're ready to turn to session 4.

You:	Did you notice any hooks showing up over the past week?
John:	Oh, plenty of hooks—hooks at work and dating hooks.
You:	So you asked Joy out?
John:	Nope. I got hooked as I went to call her, just like last week.
You:	What hook showed up this time?
John:	The thought that she's too busy and that she's probably not interested.
You:	And what five-senses information led to those?

John:	(*Laughs.*) None at all. It's all in my head.
You:	Nice noticing. You say Joy's important, so you'll find a way. How about work?
John:	You know, I'm noticing fewer hooks at work. I still have some fear of making a mistake, but I've noticed that as I speed up I've actually made fewer mistakes. It seems like I'm focusing better.
You:	That's a lot of noticing. So it sounds like you're telling me that work is progressing and dating is stuck.
John:	Yes, that sums it up well. It's funny though. I'm okay with this pace. Maybe my improved focusing at work is telling me something.
You:	That's interesting.
John:	I'm thinking that if I were to go out, I'd be in my head and not paying attention to the girl. Looking back on the few dates I've had, that was the case. I barely noticed what my dates were wearing.
You:	It sounds like you're coming up with a new toward move in regard to dating.
John:	I'm cooking up a toward move for Joy.

We'll leave John's session here. It's a small world, and you have someone named Joy in your calendar for next week, and you're wondering…

Joy

From your intake information you know that Joy is a community psychologist. She's dressed well and professionally, but maybe dressed a bit dowdily to your eye. She seems to be very physically fit but isn't showing this off. Then you notice yourself being judgmental and get back to experiencing Joy in the moment. She's very well spoken and has a lyrical voice.

When you ask Joy if you can show her the psychological flexibility point of view, she smiles and tells you she knows it well. She says she uses and presents the matrix in her work as a psychologist. Then she says she decided to see you after hearing that you also use the matrix point of view. She feels like she needs a boost in her life, and she thought reviewing the matrix with a life coach might help.

You:	I'm so glad to meet you. I think you sent someone my way.
Joy:	Oh, the guy from my stress management training? He mentioned that he wanted to move forward in life, but he didn't seem to be hunting for

psychotherapy, so I mentioned that I'd heard about a life coach who uses the matrix. I hope he came. He seemed sweet and needed a little boost.

Having established that John and Joy aren't dating and might never date, you feel okay about taking them both on as clients and proceed with the session. As a first step, you ask Joy whether the two of you can review the matrix, since it's the point of view you work from. She agrees readily and says that's what she's looking for: help with getting it out of her head and onto a piece of paper. You do your usual matrix presentation, and Joy jumps right in and engages with fresh eyes, as if she's never encountered it. The following dialogue picks up partway through that presentation.

You: And who's important to you?

Joy: *(Gets a faraway look in her eyes.)* Well, my family: Mom and Dad and my brother. I have a friend named Mae. She's also an assistant in my lab, but just part-time. She was my friend before she came to work at the lab. Mae fancies herself a matchmaker. She's a character. She's got a streak of blue in her hair and some tattoos. When I told her about the guy who came up after the presentation, she lit up. I think I'm one of her projects.

You: That's a great list. Any more?

Joy: There's a coworker named Cecil. He and I have done some research together. I've known him for years. Can I go ahead and add what's important, or am I jumping the gun?

You: Of course you can.

Joy: Work is way important. I'm one of those save-the-world types. I want my work to make a difference. My health is also important. I work out a lot and stay fit. Mae says I'm too buff and I scare guys off.

You: You certainly know how to do this. Shall we move to what shows up and gets in the way?

Joy: Well, my head gets in the way; I just think too much. I guess it's an occupational hazard, but it's funny because I show others how to get out of their heads!

You: Anything specific in that head of yours that's getting in the way?

Joy: My ego gets in the way. I'm not as good as I could be on my team. You can put ego there, or I will if you like.

You: Yes, I certainly have an ego that gets in the way at times. Here's a marker.

Joy:	And fear shows up when it comes to guys. I have no idea how to act. I intellectualize myself right out of love. Mae says I use big words that intimidate guys, and that's why they don't want to ask me out. I don't mean to. I just know a lot of words. I know fear shows up too, so I'll write that.
You:	We've gotten into your head—ego and fear, nice noticing. Does any other stuff show up and get in the way?
Joy:	That's enough for now. I know I can add more as it shows up.
You:	So what about away moves? What do you do to move away from that stuff?
Joy:	Well, I say the big words. You know, I think I might think of them and say them to move away from fear. I've never noticed that before. For ego, I act like I'm right way more than I am. I'm a woman in a man's world, so I overcompensate. I talk over others' ideas. You know, being in my head is a barrier, but it's also a value. I better put that over here too. *(Writes "in my head" in the lower right quadrant.)* Maybe it's fifty-fifty… Well, maybe sixty-forty. The older I get, the more my head is keeping me out of relationships.
You:	That's a lot of noticing. Want to head over and plan some toward moves?
Joy:	Yuck! This is tougher than I thought. I thought I knew my own matrix. Right now my head says that I'm doing plenty of toward moves already. It's a good thing I know it's bullshitting me.
You:	Where does the bullshitting go on your matrix?
Joy:	Lower left, of course. And to move away from it, I intellectualize. *(Pauses.)* To move toward at work, I'm going to keep a notebook with me and write down other people's ideas so I can be more collaborative. That's something I've been meaning to do for a while, but somehow I've managed not to.
You:	You can easily notice doing or not doing that.
Joy:	Relationships… Honestly, I left out something down here, in the lower right. I'd like to have a boyfriend, maybe get married. Maybe it's a biological clock thing. Maybe not. Anyway, having a steady boyfriend for a while is important to me.

Joy can't currently think of any relationship toward moves, so you end the session by briefly discussing hooks. As with John, you feel comfortable introducing hooks in session 1 because Joy is already familiar with the matrix. When you inquire about continuing your work together, Joy says she'd like to, so before she leaves, you invite her to notice any hooks that show up over the coming week as homework. In sessions 2 and 3, the two of you turn first to internal obstacles, and then to external barriers. When she returns for session 4, the following dialogue ensues.

You: Notice any hooks lately?

Joy: Oh my... Do you remember John? I ran into him at a coffee shop, and I got hooked in a big way.

You: What did you notice about the hook?

Joy: Fear, like crazy fear. Then I used some big words. And then my phone rang and it was my mother about my brother, and after I hung up, John had to go. I just stood there thinking that I'll never have a boyfriend. He probably thinks I'm a mess. I've been hooked for three days. Mae says I should call him, but I didn't have his number. Mae found it, but I still didn't call him.

You: Wow! That's a hook if I ever heard one.

Joy: Yes. I didn't just bite that hook; I swallowed it, and now I'm really getting pulled around. I have been writing down people's ideas at work, though. I feel foolish, but I take my notebook with me and do it.

You: You mentioned your brother. He's also in the lower right. What happened with him?

Joy: You know, I wasn't really sure about putting him down there. I don't talk about him much. He's older than me by seven years, so we sort of had separate childhoods. He's a drunk now, and we really don't talk. He asks my mom for money, but he's never asked me. She called me to fuss about him. I always listen. Strangely, I do think of him as important, but I don't see or talk to him except on holidays. We're cordial.

You: So, do you have any stories to sort?

Joy: Mae was giving me grief.

You: What was she giving you grief about?

Joy: John, of course. I didn't even remember his name. When he introduced himself again at the coffee shop, I remembered his face but not his name. Then I forgot it again after he left. Mae has a friend who works where John does, so she was able to track down his name and phone number. Anyway, she was giving me grief about not calling him.

You:	So Mae removed that external barrier of John's name and phone number for you. That's some interesting sorting. Where does John go?
Joy:	Lower right.
You:	And where does the phone number go?
Joy:	(*Pauses.*) Right now, it feels like it goes in the lower left. I want to move away from it. I know he was just being nice and saying hello. He'd think I was a weirdo if I called him out of the blue. That goes in the lower left too.
You:	Nice sorting.
Joy:	But I think about calling him anyway. He's good-looking, and Mae found out he's unattached.
You:	And where would you sort that stuff?
Joy:	The boyfriend is lower right. I guess calling might be in the upper right. But what if I blow it?
You:	And where does "What if I blow it?" go?
Joy:	Crap! Lower left.

After this session, you're a bit hooked by John and Joy's predicament. You would love to see them together. You've discussed the situation with your consultant, and staying out of it seems to be the best course. Mae seems to be on the job anyway.

Becoming a Noticing Coach

We hope that the session outline we provided in this chapter, along with the extended examples, has given you an idea of how you can use the matrix in life coaching. We also hope we've given you a good sense of the nonjudgmental and noncoercive nature of this work. One way of looking at it is that you'll serve as a noticing coach for clients. Humans have an amazing capacity to forge their own path into valued living, if they can just get out of their heads and into noticing their life as it's happening.

CHAPTER 11

Flexing the Matrix

The matrix can be integrated into other approaches. As shown in chapter 7, we have combined it with functional analytic psychotherapy to do therapeutic relationship–focused work. We've also incorporated it into a compassion-focused approach (Tirch et al., 2014). Others have used it in combination with behavioral activation, schema therapy, mindfulness training, motivational interviewing, integrative behavioral couples therapy, dialectical behavioral therapy, psychodynamic therapy, cognitive behavioral therapy, emotion-focused therapy, and, of course, more traditional ways of practicing ACT.

In this chapter, we'll review most of these integrative approaches and how they use the matrix. But first, we'll look at how the matrix's functional contextual foundations, transdiagnostic orientation, and flexibility make it a useful tool for bringing any form of therapy under appetitive control, and for assessing the success of any intervention, including the effectiveness of medications.

Bringing Therapy Under Appetitive Control

Based on everything you've read up to this point, and especially if you've started to practice some of the interventions outlined in this book, you know that matrix work focuses heavily on promoting an appetitive point of view by inviting clients to focus on choosing behaviors that involve moving toward who or what they care about. This brings the therapeutic work, the therapist's behavior, and therapy itself under appetitive control. The matrix is, at heart, a way to promote a functional contextual point of view that supports this orientation.

So when integrating the matrix with other approaches, you may find it useful to remember that what makes ACT and matrix work unique is this functional contextual point of view, not any of the specific techniques, exercises, metaphors, and so on. In its barest pragmatic essence, this point of view is about identifying and doing what works in a particular context. In the context of both life and therapy, this means identifying what the situation affords in terms of moving toward who or what is important and then choosing to do it.

There's an excellent chance that many of the things you already do in therapy and in life work in this way, helping your clients, and you, move toward who or what is important. There is no reason to discard any of that. In fact, from a functional contextual perspective, we'd advise you not to. Instead, simply experiment with combining the matrix with the parts of your approach that are already workable and effective.

Clinicians who integrate the matrix into other approaches generally report that it helps bring the entire process into a toward space that enhances clients' ability to improve their perspective-taking skills and shift their focus from an agenda centered on moving away from unpleasant experiences and engaging in unworkable behaviors. In other words, the matrix brings their therapeutic work under appetitive control.

A Measure of Intervention Success

A student we know spoke with a number of clinicians using a broad range of approaches and asked what their yardstick for a successful intervention was. He was surprised at the vagueness of many of the answers he received.

Here's our answer: Matrix work is successful when clients notice that they are better able to choose to do what's important, even in the presence of inner obstacles. To help us assess this, we've developed a brief assessment tool, the Matrix Life Dashboard, which covers four key life domains. We offer it in two forms: one that's more basic and one that uses graphics representing a car dashboard, complete with steering wheel and four dials. (Both are available for download at http://www.newharbinger.com/33605.)

No matter what intervention approach or model you're using at present, we believe that if you add this metric to your clinical work, you'll soon notice important differences in your clients and yourself. (Note that you may wish to revise the domains or add items depending on your therapeutic objective or as appropriate to specific clients.)

The Matrix Life Dashboard

Using a scale of 0 to 10, where 0 means never and 10 means nearly always, rate your current experience in each of the domains below.

I am able to choose to do what's important to me even in the presence of inner obstacles in the following domains:

Relationships: _____

Self-care and personal development: _____

Work and/or study: _____

Leisure: _____

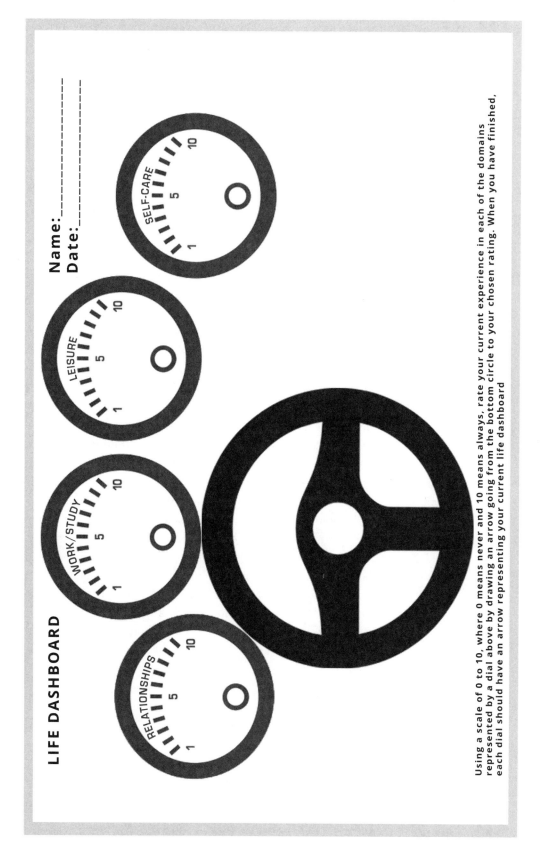

LIFE DASHBOARD

Name: _____

Date: _____

Using a scale of 0 to 10, where 0 means never and 10 means always, rate your current experience in each of the domains represented by a dial above by drawing an arrow going from the bottom circle to your chosen rating. When you have finished, each dial should have an arrow representing your current life dashboard

Using the Matrix as a Tool for Assessing the Effectiveness of Psychotropic Medications

We are psychologists and wouldn't presume to tell psychiatrists and doctors how they should prescribe to their clients. However, if you're a prescriber or a psychologist who regularly interacts with prescribers, you may be interested in how the matrix can broaden the way that clients and prescribing professionals look at symptoms and assess the effectiveness of medication regimens.

The traditional medical model largely deals with identifying symptoms and attempting to eliminate the pathogen or other underlying cause of the symptoms in order to return patients to a state of natural equilibrium. This model has given rise to the development of many successful pharmaceutical treatments for a broad range of physical ailments. When applied to mental and behavioral health, this model invites us to look for a reduction of symptoms as a yardstick for effectiveness. And because aversive inner experiences are often seen as symptoms in mental and behavioral health, psychotropic drugs generally have inner targets. Antidepressants target depressive cognitions, suicidal ideation, and feelings of despair and meaninglessness. Antianxiety medications target anxious feelings and muscular tightness (indeed, one class of anxiolytic agents, benzodiazepines, are prescribed as both antianxiety medications and muscle relaxants). Antipsychotic drugs target voices and delusions. Mood-stabilizing drugs target impulsivity and emotion dysregulation.

The underlying assumption seems to be that once these inner experiences have been dealt with and eliminated, reduced, or blunted, the person will return to equilibrium. In other words, these medications aim to reduce the frequency, intensity, or form of unwanted inner experience—the stuff in the lower left quadrant of the matrix. The SUDs acronym—subjective units of distress—which is so often used in these contexts, pretty much encapsulates the approach: prescribe a medication and regularly measure SUDs levels. While there's nothing terribly wrong with measuring SUDs, doing so without considering other criteria may reinforce the functional importance of SUDs for patients and clinicians alike and contribute to stuck loops. Plus, it may feed dependence on psychotropic drugs. Indeed, when patients try to taper off of these drugs, many of them experience an increase in SUDs, often resulting in a resumption of prescription.

Here's a dialogue that illustrates the consequences this focus on SUDs can have. It was provided by a colleague, an MD, who reported that he'd had many such conversations before bringing the matrix into his work.

MD: How have you been doing since I prescribed the pain medication?

Patient: The pain is a little better, but it's still there.

MD: Okay. So where would you evaluate your pain on that SUDs scale of 0 to 10, measuring subjective units of distress? I see here your pain was at 9 last time. And now where is it?

Patient: Well, it's still there, but less strong I guess, so maybe between 7 and 8.

MD: Okay, and have you been able to get out of bed and do stuff around the house?

Patient: Yes, but the pain is still there.

MD: Okay. And have you been able to go out for walks?

Patient: Yes, but the pain is still there.

And so on… This type of conversation reflects a context that's so geared toward reduction of SUDs that patients—and doctors—might easily miss potential improvements in other areas of life. An alternative would be also asking whether patients are more able to choose behaviors that help them move toward who and what they care about—a valued life with more purpose and meaning. This can be done in a complementary way, in tandem with measuring SUDs, as illustrated in the following dialogue (in which the MD is using a rough, hand-drawn matrix).

MD: So, you're feeling depressed down here (*pointing at the bottom left quadrant*), with dark thoughts, despair, sadness, worries about the future, and all the painful stuff that shows up. On a scale of 0 to 10, how would you rate your present level of distress on an average day?

Patient: Close to 8.5.

MD: Okay. And up here (*pointing at the top right quadrant*), how would you rate your level of actions to move toward who or what is important to you? I mean things that I or someone else could see you do. Again on a scale of 0 to 10, with 0 being none and 10 being as many actions as you could hope to do in twenty-four hours, where would you be on that scale on an average day?

Patient: Oh my… I'm so depressed these days. It's pretty low. I'd say around 2.

MD: Okay. So here's what we're going to do: I'm going to prescribe this medication and ask you to come back for a follow-up in a few weeks. During that appointment we'll look at these two scales again. The medication may have an impact on reducing the painful stuff down there (*pointing at the bottom left quadrant*), but really it's aimed as much, if not more, toward helping you do more of this up here (*pointing at the top right quadrant*). See if you can keep track of both scales, maybe by recording your ratings at the end of each day, using an average for your SUDs over the course of the day. Would you be willing to do that?

When the patient comes back, the doctor could either ask for both his SUDs and toward moves ratings since their previous appointment, or simply ask for an on-the-spot rating. If toward moves have increased, treatment has worked, regardless of SUDs ratings. If SUDs ratings have decreased but so have toward moves, it may be a good idea to rethink or adjust the prescription. In any case, treatment will have a greater focus on toward moves, and therefore the patient will too, which may serve to promote toward moves in the long run.

Throwing the Matrix into the Mix

As mentioned at the beginning of this chapter, many clinicians have integrated the matrix into other approaches, and they often notice that their clients subsequently become more engaged in therapy. They also notice that they find their work more fun and satisfying. We'll turn to those integrative approaches shortly, but first we want to address what may seem a fine point of terminology.

Throughout this book, we've largely used the terms "hooks" and "getting hooked" to describe how inner experience can drag people off course, pulling them into behaving differently than the person they want to be. Of course, we are well aware that other approaches use different terminology for what we've referred to as hooks and getting hooked. Among these other names you'll find maladaptive early schemas, cognitive distortions, unconscious defense mechanisms, cognitive fusion, and experiential avoidance.

While we've found that the term "hooks" works well for most clients, don't let it hook you. Again, this is about function, not form. One key aspect of matrix work is to help clients notice the function of their inner experience (Does it promote away or toward moves?) and of their behavior (Are they moving toward who or what is important or away from inner stuff that shows up and gets in the way?). If other terms work better for you, use them. This applies to all the topographical aspects of matrix work. Do what's effective for you in helping clients do what's effective for them.

As long as you keep your work in a functional contextual framework (as we'll describe at the end of this chapter) there is no end (that we know of, anyway) to the integrative power of the matrix. If, however, you lose sight of this perspective, you run the risk of using the matrix as a tool for attempting to change clients' thoughts, emotions, and feelings—thereby reinforcing the functional importance of thoughts, emotions, and feelings. This work is always about helping clients become better able to choose to move toward who or what is important to them, even in the presence of inner obstacles.

The Matrix and Behavioral Activation

Fabian Olaz has developed a simple protocol for integrating matrix work into behavioral activation. His approach makes use of the Matrix Activity Log, which we include here (it's also available for download at http://www.newharbinger.com/33605). The basics of the approach are to work through steps 1 through 4, as described in part 1 of this book, while inviting clients to use the worksheet to record their behavior throughout the day. To promote recording this information frequently, the worksheet is divided into hourly slots.

MATRIX ACTIVITY LOG

Name : _____   Dates : from _____ to _____

Day						
6–7 a.m.						
7–8 a.m.						
8–9 a.m.						
9–10 a.m.						
10–11 a.m.						
11–12 p.m.						
12–1 p.m.						
1–2 p.m.						
2–3 p.m.						
3–4 p.m.						
4–5 p.m.						
5–6 p.m.						
6–7 p.m.						
7–8 p.m.						
8–9 p.m.						
9–10 p.m.						
10–11 p.m.						

For each action you note on the sheet, add an A if you noticed it as an away move and a T if as a toward move. For toward moves, add * if it was easy to engage, ** if it was moderately difficult, and *** if it was very difficult to engage.

Noticing toward and away moves as many times a day as possible activates one of the two main discriminations of matrix work and tends to increase noticing toward moves. Rating the difficulty of engaging in toward moves ensures that clients will appreciate their efforts, thus increasing the chances they'll continue engaging in difficult toward moves. In technical terms, this rating activates augmentals, increasing the reinforcing functions of engaging in difficult toward moves. The protocol includes simple activities that blend activation tasks, mindfulness, values, and work on identifying which situations and environments promote engaging in toward moves (see Kanter, Busch, & Rusch, 2009).

The Matrix and Schema Therapy

Over the years, a number of clinicians have integrated schema therapy and ACT. The matrix has joined the party and is now used to help clients sort their schemas and modes of responding to them when each is activated. Schemas are often—but not always—sorted in the bottom left quadrant, while specific ways of responding to them are sorted as either toward or away moves, depending on their function. Schemas and modes of responding can provide useful shorthand for common hooks and ways of biting, respectively. They can also provide additional structure, which some clinicians and clients find helpful.

The Matrix and Mindfulness Training

As discussed in the introduction, the matrix is a powerful tool for training mindfulness without formal practice. This quality also makes it well suited to integration with mindfulness training. Once people have learned the basics of meditation, they can engage in focused practice around noticing the difference between five-senses and mental experience. Then you can invite them to work through what is important to them, the hooks that can show up and get in the way, and how these can result in living on autopilot.

A number of mindfulness trainers have reported that the matrix can serve as the next logical step after mindfulness meditation training. Many people wonder what to do once they've learned to mindfully observe their passing thoughts and emotions. Introducing the right-hand side of the matrix can bring a more pragmatic focus, helping people find their own solutions by applying mindfulness skills in everyday life in the service of moving toward their values.

The Matrix and Motivational Interviewing

If you're familiar with motivational interviewing (Miller & Rollnick, 1991), you may have noticed that the therapist stance we aim for, in particular through yessing, shares a lot with the motivational interviewing stance of rolling with resistance. Another commonality stems from the horizontal axis of the matrix. Encouraging clients to notice both sides of the matrix—toward and away—reflects the motivational interviewing approach of inviting clients to notice the advantages and disadvantages of continuing or changing their present behavior. Interestingly, a number of motivational interviewing clinicians have told us that using the matrix feels more flexible than asking clients to rate advantages and disadvantages.

The Matrix and Integrative Behavioral Couples Therapy

Integrative behavioral couples therapy (Jacobson & Christensen, 1996) is an empirically based approach that is effective in couples work. It focuses on identifying the broad themes of a couple's conflicts to illuminate which parts of the couple's difficulties arise from deep-set differences. These can then be targeted for reconciliation through acceptance so that the couple can establish more effective communication and deeper intimacy. Matrix couples work is described in some detail in chapter 9 of this book, and the approach there can be seamlessly integrated with integrative behavioral couples therapy, with the matrix aiding in swift identification of couples' stuck loops. The matrix point of view also provides couples with a distanced way of talking about their hot-button issues.

The Matrix and Dialectical Behavior Therapy

Dialectical behavior therapy (DBT; Linehan, 1993) is a psychotherapy developed to work with clients who have emotional regulation problems, especially those diagnosed with borderline personality disorder. These clients show great reactivity to emotional stimuli and a high degree of instability in their sense of self. From an ACT perspective, they often display overgeneralized experiential avoidance, serious deictic framing difficulties, and complications with identifying values—deficits that also give rise to serious obstacles to empathy and valued action when these clients experience invalidation. The matrix is starting to influence DBT practitioners and approaches (Reyes, Vargas, & Tena, 2015). Some DBT therapists include it as part of their skills training work with clients, and others use it as an integrative model to organize their DBT work and conduct functional analyses (aka chain analysis in DBT). Matrix work is a useful way to train psychological flexibility with these clients because it allows them to notice and contact their behaviors—both public and private—and helps them understand the functions that govern those behaviors in a less threatening way.

DBT work is usually done in four stages. During pretreatment and stage 1, the matrix can be a useful tool for motivating clients to buy in to treatment and reduce problem behaviors, which, with these clients at this stage, can sabotage therapy (therapy-interfering behaviors) and may even be life-threatening (life-interfering behaviors). Increasing mindfulness is a goal of stage 1, and the matrix, with its emphasis on noticing, is a great tool for promoting this. Stage 2 generally focuses on working with PTSD, and given that the matrix was initially developed for this very purpose, it's well suited to this work (see Polk & Burkhart, 2014). Stage 3 involves working through difficulties in everyday life, and stage 4 turns to helping clients overcome feelings of inadequacy and build a capacity for joy. The matrix fits perfectly with these goals, since it emphasizes working with values and building a life filled with meaning and vitality.

The Matrix and Psychodynamic Approaches

Psychodynamic approaches often focus on exploring clients' early life experiences to arrive at interpretations of how the experiences have come to influence present-day motivations and behavior. In our trainings and in the worldwide ACT community, we've met a number of clinicians who report that the matrix complements this approach by facilitating psychodynamically coherent sorting.

Those who have incorporated the matrix into psychodynamic interventions report that they generally see faster change in clients. This may be because the matrix shifts how both therapists and clients relate to psychodynamically informed interpretation, turning the focus from finding the "right" interpretation to finding one that not only makes sense of the past but also works to help clients move forward in the present and illuminates the future. Furthermore, the matrix aids both clients and clinicians in focusing on and measuring meaningful change in the present, so both are less governed by the shadows of the past.

The Matrix and CBT

Clinicians in Mexico have reported using the matrix as a way to both train and apply CBT (Reyes & Vargas, in press). To a large extent, this application of the matrix depends on how you conceive of using CBT. With the matrix, you can effectively work on reducing anxiety or on modifying cognitions, as long as this is done in the service of making it easier for clients to engage in toward moves, even in the presence of difficult cognitions and emotions.

As one example, you can ask clients to notice where their thoughts show up in the matrix and then help them look for evidence that a given thought is a description of the world of five senses, versus a generalization that their minds have abstracted from past experience or even other thoughts. Then you can engage them in recognizing their cognitive distortions and what they do next in a way similar to working with hooks.

Integrating the Matrix with Traditional ACT

This may seem like a strange section, given that the matrix is all ACT all the time. However, we include traditional ACT here because many ACT therapists are using the matrix as part of a more traditional ACT approach. Some use the matrix for setting up the point of view, then address the six facets of the hexaflex model of psychological flexibility. Others tend to use the matrix in the background, rather than with clients, to help them track where they or their clients are at any given time, or as a tool for case conceptualization (Schoendorff, 2014). The matrix can thus be used as a primary vehicle for delivering ACT or as one part of a broader array of ACT strategies.

When first exposed to the matrix, many ACT practitioners have a hard time believing that such a simple diagram, training two basic discriminations, can accomplish most of the work in ACT. However, after initially using the matrix in limited ways, some of these same practitioners gradually discover the power of the diagram and begin using it more regularly.

If you take your time with the matrix and take a deeper look at the RFT-based processes the matrix brings into play (as discussed in this book and in Schoendorff et al., 2014), you may come to see, as we have, that these two lines on a piece of paper capture the heart of what ACT is about. Of course, should you elect to become a matrix practitioner, we recommend that you read at least one of the traditional ACT books, such as *Acceptance and Commitment Therapy: The Process and Practice of Mindful Change* (Hayes, Strosahl, & Wilson, 2012), or *Mindfulness for Two: An Acceptance and Commitment Therapy Approach to Mindfulness in Psychotherapy* (Wilson, 2008). Doing so will ensure that your approach is informed by the full ACT model. In addition, you'll undoubtedly find useful ways of thinking about your clinical work and many effective exercises and metaphors that you can integrate into your matrix work.

Functional Contextualism to Bring Them All Together

We believe that the integrative power of the matrix, suggested by the material in this chapter, comes from the functional contextualist foundations that undergird it. Functional contextualism is the cement that can ensure a strong and coherent foundation for integrating the matrix into many therapeutic approaches. At root, functional contextualism is just a way of looking at the world—a radically pragmatic point of view that eschews seeking answers to questions about the nature of things in favor of seeking to identify what works in relation to chosen goals. Ultimately, such questions can never be fully answered absent a context. This has profound implications in relation to the nature of scientific endeavors. On a less grand scale, it is immensely important for effective interventions and clinical work. For example, instead of asking, "Is the thought 'I can never do this' realistic?" a functional contextual approach to the question is whether that thought works to help you get where you want to go or behave like the person you want to be. Depending on the context, it may or it may not.

In terms of clinical work, one of the biggest benefits a functional contextual approach delivers is freeing conversations from the futile pursuit of determining what's real and what isn't. After all, if the brightest philosophers have made little progress in answering this question over the past four thousand years, what are the chances we can do better? Therefore, we choose to engage in conversations about noticing what works and what doesn't, and in which contexts.

Conclusion

It has been our great pleasure to write *The Essential Guide to the ACT Matrix*. Because the matrix is so rich, there is much more we wish we could have included in these pages. And just like ACT, the matrix is a fully transdiagnostic approach, so we haven't gone into the details of using it with particular clinical presentations. This may well be the subject of future books—perhaps written by you as you become adept at using the matrix with your own clients.

As we've stressed throughout this book, the key to using the matrix is to practice using it. Once you get your basic moves down, go beyond what we've shown you to see where and how the matrix fits into your practice and your life in general. You will undoubtedly find new places to use it and new uses for it. We know this because the matrix was designed to increase psychological flexibility, which leads to creating new behaviors. So as you use it, you will have moments of insight along the lines of "Gee, I could use the matrix to do X." Go with these insights and try them out. The only limit is your imagination. And if you find a creative, new way to use the matrix, let us know; we'd love to hear about it.

The people you work with who also use the matrix—colleagues and clients alike—will have similar insights about new ways they can use the matrix. Jump up and down with glee (or at least look excited) when this happens. These are precious moments in which the human mind is deriving new stuff. We never tire of watching people gaining a greater awareness of the big picture of their lives and then developing creative new ways to live life to the fullest.

In your journey with the matrix, people will probably ask you, "What is this matrix?" We often respond along these lines: "The matrix is a diagram of a human being a human. In order to see the human being human, we ask questions with deep respect. Then we carefully notice what shows up after we ask those respectful questions. As we fill in the diagram, the stuff of being human becomes clearer—often clear enough to help people find workable behaviors for the ongoing task of living a valued life." As you bring the matrix into your work and into your life, you'll soon come up with your own ways of answering this question.

Being a human is often tough, and we all get stuck. The matrix can help anyone loosen up and find a way back into valued living. All of us sometimes blame others or circumstances for the fact that we're stuck; that's also very human. Using the matrix, we can notice that blaming and its unworkability and get back to increasing psychological flexibility.

We made the choice to devote the second part of this book to using the matrix in the social world because we believe relationships and community are at the heart of the human experience and what's important to us as humans. It is no accident that the question "Who is important?" is the pivot around which matrix work turns. We encourage you not only to bring the matrix into your relationships and communities, but also to join the wider ACT community (http://www.contextualscience.org), where you can become part of shaping the change we all need.

We also hope that, through this book, the matrix can contribute to spreading functional contextualism and acceptance and commitment therapy to more people, groups, and communities. We wish for this not because we are particularly attached to names, approaches, or labels, but because as humans we all need a psychology that can better meet the challenges of being human: a psychology that serves to help everyone—individuals, groups, and communities—get unstuck and move toward who or what is most deeply important to us as a beautiful and fragile species sharing this wondrous and precious planet.

Acknowledgments

I first would like to thank my dear wife and colleague Marie-France for her support and love, and for all the great ideas she contributed to this book and to my training work more generally. I want to acknowledge the contribution of my cowriters, Kevin, Mark, and Fabi. It's been a joy working with you, friends! Thanks to Carlos Rivera for his help with chapter 8. A huge thank you to Tom Szabo for checking the technical RFT stuff throughout the book. Any remaining mistakes are entirely our responsibility.

Jasmine Star, our copy editor, was a privilege to work with. I learned so much from her. Copyediting does not get better than this. Thank you, Tesilya Hanauer and New Harbinger, for believing in this project. Thank you, Timothy Gordon for support and some great ideas about working with kids. Thank you, Lisa Coyne and Darin Cairns for inspiring some of the children and parenting parts of this book. Thanks to all the clients and participants in my workshops who have shaped the six steps approach. Thank you, matrix practitioners who have shared how you use the matrix with different populations and integrate it with other approaches. There are many of you and some I am afraid I'll forget: Susan Chapel, Jana Grand, Thomas Holmes, Paulo Quintero, Rob Purssey, Michel Reyes, and Sheri Turrell. Huge thanks to Michel Reyes, Nathalia Vargas, Michael Levin, Ben Pierce, and Sarah Potts for conducting research in using the matrix, and thank you Kieron O'Connor for letting me integrate the matrix into my own ACT research. Thank you Troy DuFrene and Praxis for integrating the matrix in the ACT Boot Camp trainings. Thank you Enya Tougas and all our volunteers at the Contextual Psychology Institute.

Finally, I want to dedicate this book to the people I have hurt in the past when I was stuck in trying to move away from my suffering rather than moving toward who and what is truly important. I wish I could have behaved differently and more lovingly then, and will continue working at it, at moving toward repairing, loving, and making myself useful.

—Benjamin Schoendorff

Thank you to my loving family. To my dear wife, Mary Alyce Burkhart. Her support, love, and matrix insights are ingrained in the pages of this book. To my daughter Ellie, who has taken the matrix to her graduate studies in psychology. To my daughter Lizzy, who has taken the matrix into her high school and her work with animals. To my son Brendan, who shows how he uses the matrix every day. To Pat and Dwight Keene and Galen Moore, for being such good friends.

Thanks also... To Jerold Hambright who has spent thousands of hours playing ACT like jazz with me. To Benji Schoendorff and his tireless devotion to writing and editing. To Mark Webster and his passion for making the matrix a trainable skill. To Fabián Olaz, who reminds us all that it's all about showing each other the way to peace, love, and understanding. To Phil Tenaglia for getting the matrix into schools. To Steve Hayes and Kelly Wilson for their openness and support. To David Sloan Wilson for helping connect the matrix to evolution science. To Adriana Zilberman and Mara Lins for their loving support in Brazil and Argentina. To New Harbinger Publications for accepting and then nurturing this project. A huge thanks to Jasmine Star for her expert copy editing. And thanks to everyone willing to pick up the matrix and give it a try. Thank you.

—Kevin Polk

I first would like to thank Benji, my friend and master for inviting me to be part of this amazing project and for being my buddy in my new way of living life. To Kevin and Mark, for opening the "matrix door" and welcoming me as part of the matrix team. To Jerold Hambright, a wise and generous man who taught me about the matrix, but more important still, taught me about humility and kindness. Thank you to Yanina Alladio for the ideas about and collaboration in working with kids; you are an amazing and inspiring professional. Thanks to Tesilya Hanauer and the team at New Harbinger Publications for a fantastic job.

I have to say thanks to all the ACT community, especially to those who trained me and gave me confidence about my way of doing and training ACT (in no particular order): Benji Schoendorff, Kevin Polk, Mark Webster, Jerold Hambright, Vijay Shankar, Chris McCurry, Steve Hayes, Kelly Wilson, Kirk Strosahl, Patti Robinson, Matt Villatte, Carmen Luciano, Niklas Törneke, and Robyn Walser.

Thanks to all my clients and to the participants in my workshops and courses, from Argentina, Brazil, Peru, and Chile. Your respect, love, and confidence move me toward the right side of my matrix when hooks show up.

Thanks to my team at the Integral Center of Contextual Psychotherapies, in Córdoba (Argentina), and my colleagues in Argentina who taught me to be aware of the contingencies of my behavior. Thanks to my students at the Faculty of Psychology at the National University of Córdoba for the looks on your faces when you're learning, which remind me why I chose this profession.

This book is especially dedicated to my dear wife Gabriela, and my two pretty princesses Pía and Malena. Your love and company is the "best excuse" for me to try to be a better man, day after day. Thanks to my siblings and my parents, for being a model of persistence and willingness.

Those who know me know that participating in this book is a dream come true for me. And although my mind is still telling me that I don't deserve it, now I can notice that and keep on moving myself toward what is really important in my life, thanks to this fantastic model, which has made my life a little bit simpler.

—Fabian Olaz

Thanks goes to Kevin Polk for having the ideas that started this process, and for inviting me over to the VA's Togus Regional Benefit Office. Thanks to Jerold Hambright, whose contribution is less visible. Thanks to Benji for his hard work with the writing and to Fabián for his enthusiasm and support. Thanks to the team at New Harbinger Publications for pulling the work together into a clear structure.

Thanks to all the clients and colleagues who participated in the development of these ideas. You have been the greatest teachers and it is your experience that shaped the matrix into the simple format in which it exists today. Finally, I am grateful to my wife and family, who have allowed me the time and space to let these ideas flourish. I truly appreciate all your support.

—Mark Webster

References

Aurelius, M. (1964). *Meditations* (M. Staniforth, Trans.). Baltimore: Penguin.

Bargh, J. A., Chen, M., & Burrows, L. (1996). Automaticity of social behavior: Direct effects of trait construct and stereotype activation on action. *Journal of Personality and Social Psychology 71*(2), 230–244.

Biglan, A. (2015). *The nurture effect: How the science of human behavior can improve our lives and our world.* Oakland, CA: New Harbinger.

Callaghan, G. M. (2001). *Functional Idiographic Assessment Template (FIAT).* Unpublished manual, San Jose State University.

Callaghan, G. M. (2006). The Functional Idiographic Assessment Template (FIAT) system. *Behavior Analyst Today 7*(3): 357–398.

Cioffi, D., & Holloway, J. (1993). Delayed costs of suppressed pain. *Journal of Personality and Social Psychology 64*(2), 274–282.

Cordova, J. V., & Scott, R. L. (2001). Intimacy: A behavioral interpretation. *Behavior Analyst 24*(1): 75–86.

Coyne, L. W., & Murrell, A. R. (2009). *The joy of parenting: An acceptance and commitment therapy guide to effective parenting in the early years.* Oakland, CA: New Harbinger.

Darrow, S. M., Callaghan, G. C., Bonow, J. T., & Follette, W. C. (2014). The Functional Idiographic Assessment Template—Questionnaire (FIAT-Q): Initial psychometric properties. *Journal of Contextual Behavioral Science 3*(2): 124–135.

Gottman, J. (1997). *The heart of parenting: Raising an emotionally intelligent child.* New York: Simon and Schuster.

Hayes, S. C. (with Smith, S.). (2005). *Get out of your mind and into your life: The new acceptance and commitment therapy.* Oakland, CA: New Harbinger.

Hayes, S. C., Strosahl, K. D., Bunting, K., Twohig, M., & Wilson, K. G. (2004). What is acceptance and commitment therapy? In S. C. Hayes & K. D. Strosahl (Eds.), *A practical guide to acceptance and commitment therapy.* New York: Springer.

Hayes, S. C., Strosahl, K. D., & Wilson, K. G. (1999). *Acceptance and commitment therapy: An experiential approach to behavior change.* New York: Guilford.

Hayes, S. C., Strosahl, K. D., & Wilson, K. G. (2012). *Acceptance and commitment therapy: The process and practice of mindful change,* second edition. New York: Guilford.

Holt-Lunstad, J., Smith, T. B., & Layton, J. B. (2010). Social relationships and mortality risk: A meta-analytic review. *PLoS Medicine* 7(7): e1000316.

Jacobson, N. S., & Christensen, A. (1996). *Acceptance and change in couple therapy: A therapist's guide to transforming relationships.* New York: Norton.

Kabat-Zinn, J. (1994). *Wherever you go, there you are: Mindfulness meditation in everyday life.* New York: Hyperion.

Kanter, J., Busch, A., & Rusch, L. (2009). *Behavioral activation: Distinctive features.* New York: Routledge.

Kazdin, A. E. (2005). *Parent management training: Treatment for oppositional, aggressive, and antisocial behavior in children and adolescents.* Oxford: Oxford University Press.

Kazdin, A. E., & Rotella, C. (2013). *The everyday parenting toolkit: The Kazdin method for easy, step-by-step, lasting change for you and your child.* New York: Houghton Mifflin Harcourt.

Koerner, K. (2012). *Doing dialectical behavior therapy: A practical guide.* New York: Guilford.

Kohlenberg, R. J., & Tsai, M. (1991). *Functional analytic psychotherapy.* New York: Springer.

Linehan, M. M. (1993). *Cognitive-behavioral treatment of borderline personality disorder.* New York: Guilford.

Linehan, M. M. (1997). Validation and psychotherapy. In A. Bohart & L. Greenberg (Eds.), *Empathy reconsidered: New directions in psychotherapy.* Washington, DC: American Psychological Association.

McCurry, C. (2009). *Parenting your anxious child with mindfulness and acceptance: A powerful new approach to overcoming fear, panic, and worry using acceptance and commitment therapy.* Oakland, CA: New Harbinger.

McHugh, L., & Stewart, I. (Eds.). (2012). *The self and perspective taking: Contributions and applications from modern behavioral science.* Oakland, CA: New Harbinger.

Miller, W. R., & Rollnick, S. (1991). *Motivational interviewing: Preparing people for change.* New York: Guilford.

Polk, K. L. (2014). The matrix, evolution, and improving work-group functioning with Ostrom's eight design principles. In K. L. Polk & B. Schoendorff (Eds.), *The ACT matrix: A new approach to building psychological flexibility across settings and populations.* Oakland, CA: New Harbinger.

Polk, K. L., & Burkhart, M. A. (2014). Something you can never forget: The matrix and PTSD. In K. Polk & B. Schoendorff (Eds.), *The ACT matrix: A new approach to building psychological flexibility across settings and populations.* Oakland, CA: New Harbinger.

Polk, K. L., & Schoendorff, B. (Eds.) (2014). *The ACT matrix: A new approach to building psychological flexibility across settings and populations.* Oakland, CA: New Harbinger.

Rehfeldt, R. A., & Barnes-Holmes, Y. (2009). *Derived relational responding applications for learners with autism and other developmental disabilities: A progressive guide to change.* Oakland, CA: New Harbinger.

Reyes, M. (2015, July). "How" is important: The matrix as functional analytic psychotherapy rule 5 and CRB evoking tool. In B. Schoendorff (Chair), *Working the matrix on interpersonal settings: Building empathy, pro-sociability, and ACL.* Symposium conducted at the Association for Contextual Behavioral Science World Conference 13, Berlin, Germany.

Reyes, M. & Vargas, A. N. (in press). Desarrollo de la terapia conductual contextual en México. In O. Rodrigues (Comp.), *Historia del Conductismo en Latinoamérica.* São Paulo: Asociación Latinoamericana de Modificación de Conducta.

Reyes, M., Vargas, N., & Miranda, E. (2015, July). Comparison of 4 brief contextual behavioral interventions for borderline personality disorder: The process of building an empirically supported treatment as usual. In K. Strosahl (Chair), *Brief ACT interventions: Understanding their benefit and processes of change.* Symposium conducted at the Association for Contextual Behavioral Science World Conference 13, Berlin, Germany.

Reyes, M. A., Vargas, A. N., & Tena, A. (2015). Hacia un modelo teórico del trastorno límite de la personalidad. *Psicología Iberoamericana, 23*(2), 66–76.

Rother, M. (2010). *Toyota kata: Managing people for improvement, adaptiveness, and superior results.* New York: McGraw-Hill.

Sandoz, E., Wilson, K. G., & DuFrene, T. (2011). *Acceptance and commitment therapy for eating disorders: A process-focused guide to treating anorexia and bulimia.* Oakland, CA: New Harbinger.

Schoendorff, B. (2014). Casing the matrix: A tool for case conceptualization. In K. Polk & B. Schoendorff (Eds.), *The ACT matrix: A new approach to building psychological flexibility across settings and populations.* Oakland, CA: New Harbinger.

Schoendorff, B., & Bolduc, M. F. (2014). You, me, and the matrix: A guide to relationship-oriented ACT. In K. Polk & B. Schoendorff (Eds.), *The ACT matrix: A new approach to building psychological flexibility across settings and populations.* Oakland, CA: New Harbinger.

Schoendorff, B., Grand, J., & Bolduc, M. F. (2011). *La thérapie d'acceptation et d'engagement: guide clinique.* Brussels: DeBoeck.

Schoendorff, B., Purcell-Lalonde, M., & O'Connor, K. (2013). Les thérapies de troisième vague dans le traitement du trouble obsessionnel-compulsif: Application de la thérapie d'acceptation et d'engagement [Third-wave therapies in the treatment of obsessive-compulsive disorder: Applying acceptance and commitment therapy]. *Santé mentale au Québec* 38(2): 153–173.

Schoendorff, B., Webster, M., & Polk, K. L. (2014). Under the hood: Basic processes underlying the matrix. In K. L. Polk & B. Schoendorff (Eds.), *The ACT matrix: A new approach to building psychological flexibility across settings and populations.* Oakland, CA: New Harbinger.

Seys, A. (2014). In business: The matrix for team building and professional stress. In K. L. Polk & B. Schoendorff (Eds.), *The ACT matrix: A new approach to building psychological flexibility across settings and populations.* Oakland, CA: New Harbinger.

Tirch, D., Schoendorff, B., & Silberstein, L. R. (2014). *The ACT practitioner's guide to the science of compassion: Tools for fostering psychological flexibility.* Oakland, CA: New Harbinger.

Törneke, N. (2010). *Learning RFT: An introduction to relational frame theory and its clinical applications.* Oakland, CA: New Harbinger.

Tsai, M., Kohlenberg, R. J., Kanter, J. W., Kohlenberg, B., Follette, W. C., & Callaghan, G. M. (Eds.). (2009). *A guide to functional analytic psychotherapy: Awareness, courage, love, and behaviorism.* New York: Springer.

Wegner, D. M., Ansfield, M., & Pilloff, D. (1998). The putt and the pendulum: Ironic effects of the mental control of action. *Psychological Science* 9(3): 196–199.

Wegner, D. M., Schneider, D. J., Carter, S. R., & White, T. L. (1987). Paradoxical effects of thought suppression. *Journal of Personal and Social Psychology* 53(1): 5–13.

Wenzlaff, R. M., & Wegner, D. M. (2000). Thought suppression. *Annual Review of Psychology* 51, 59–91.

Wilson, K. G. (with DuFrene, T.). (2008). *Mindfulness for two: An acceptance and commitment therapy approach to mindfulness in psychotherapy.* Oakland, CA: New Harbinger.

Kevin L. Polk, PhD, is a clinical psychologist who has been a practicing for twenty-six years, primarily helping veterans and others with troubling trauma memories. For the past eleven years, he has dedicated himself to the study of acceptance and commitment therapy (ACT)—spending close to 27,000 hours studying the philosophy and theory behind ACT, and learning and designing ACT interventions. He is a peer-reviewed ACT trainer who is passionate about teaching others how to use the ACT Matrix to increase psychological flexibility and valued living. Find out more at www.drkevinpolk.com.

Benjamin Schoendorff, MA, MSc, is director of the Contextual Psychology Institute in Montreal, QC, Canada. He is involved in ACT research at the Montreal University Mental Health Institute, and a clinical psychologist in private practice working with adults, children, teens, and couples. Schoendorff is passionate about making ACT simple for both therapists and clients. He's authored and coauthored several ACT books in French, coedited *The ACT Matrix* with Kevin Polk, and coauthored *The ACT Practitioner's Guide to the Science of Compassion* with Dennis Tirch and Laura Silberstein. A peer-reviewed ACT trainer and certified functional analytic psychotherapy (FAP) trainer, Schoendorff has led approximately two-hundred workshops around the world, and is currently disseminating the six-step ACT Matrix approach at the heart of this book. His workshops are widely appreciated for their direct clinical applicability, deep humanity, and warm sense of humor. In his spare time, Schoendorff loves travelling with his wife and young son Thomas, and sharing his love for ACT and the Matrix. Find out more at www.contextpsy.com.

Mark Webster is a registered psychotherapist with the United Kingdom Council for Psychotherapy (UKCP). Following a first career in the computer industry, he worked for ten years at a specialist personality disorder clinic in the National Health Service (NHS). His involvement in third-wave cognitive behavioral therapy (CBT) began with dialectical behavior therapy (DBT) in 1997, which led to an early interest in ACT. Webster has been an ACT trainer since 2002, and currently runs his own business specializing in acceptance and mindfulness therapies. In 2005, he founded the ACT special interest group within the British Association for Behavioural and Cognitive Psychotherapies (BABCP). In 2008, with Kevin Polk, he created the ACT Matrix, a very user-friendly way of delivering ACT in a group setting. Webster's main interest is in finding ways to make ACT more widely available outside of traditional mental health settings. He has recently founded a community interest company called ACT Peer Recovery CIC to develop peer recovery in addiction and mental health. In addition to offering training in mental health, he regularly conducts ACT workshops for physical health practitioners, including nurses, physiotherapists, and occupational therapists. Webster has been practicing mindfulness for over twenty-five years, and is current chair of the UKCP's Cognitive Psychotherapies College.

Fabian O. Olaz, PsyD, is adjunct professor in clinical psychology and psychotherapies, and researcher and director of the Interpersonal Behavior Laboratory in the faculty of psychology at the National University of Córdoba in Argentina. He is an ACT and functional analytic psychotherapy supervisor and psychotherapist at the Integral Center of Contextual Psychotherapy (CIPCO), and a recognized trainer in Argentina, Brazil, and other South American countries.

Index

derived relational responding, 10

Derived Relational Responding (Rehfeldt and Barnes-Holmes), 4

dialectical behavior therapy (DBT), 251–252

Differences Detective game, 205–206

discriminations, 152–153

E

emotional coaching, 188

emotions: clients claiming to control, 79–80, 81–82; cognitive control efforts and, 82–83; parenting principle of validating, 196–197; teenagers and, 200–201. *See also* inner experiences

empathy, 145, 182, 195

empty chair work, 143

ending treatment, 111, 147

Everyday Parenting Toolkit, The (Kazdin and Rotella), 190

experience: broadening awareness of, 59–60; five senses vs. mental, 2; matrix work related to, 35; sorting on the matrix, 4–5; validation of, 90

experience line, 2

experiential exercises: for children, 205–208; Mother Cat Exercise, 114–119; settling-in noticing exercise, 42–43

explaining vs. pointing, 31

external barriers, 231–233

F

FAP. *See* functional analytic psychotherapy

feeling good trap, 106

first-name perspective, 146–147

five-senses experiences: mental experiences vs., 2; sorting inner experiences and, 70–72

flexible framing, 11

flexible tracking, 109, 125, 128

Ford, Henry, 234

framing: away moves, 61–62; control efforts, 85; deictic, 37–38, 85, 144–147; hierarchical, 38; hooks, 85; perspective-taking and, 144–147; rule following and, 126; teaching flexible, 11, 37–38; temporal, 61; verbal aikido and, 109–110

functional analytic psychotherapy (FAP), 157; awareness, courage, and love in, 166–169; clinically relevant behaviors and, 162; FAP Session Bridging Form, 176; five rules of, 169–170

functional contextualism, 4, 15–16, 35, 41, 151, 243, 253

fusion, 83, 84

future stuck situations, 137, 142–143

G

goofiness in dialogues, 142

Gordon, Timothy, 185

Gottman, John, 188, 190, 196

green belt validation, 91–92

H

Hambright, Jerold, 4

Heart of Parenting: Raising an Emotionally Intelligent Child, The (Gottman), 190

here-now perspective, 139, 140, 141

hexaflex in ACT, 4, 7

hierarchical framing, 38

high-probability behaviors, 194–195

holding ideas lightly, 36–37

home practice, 29–30; life coaching and, 227; Mother Cat Exercise as, 119; noticing and working with hooks as, 79; noticing toward or away moves as, 30, 54, 137–138; perspective taking as,

137–138; presenting to teens, 201; verbal aikido as, 104

hooks, 72–79; alternative terms for, 248; catch-and-release example of, 77–78; children and, 205; content-related, 140; couples work and, 217; defusion work and, 84–85; home practice of noticing, 79; introducing to clients, 72–74; potential traps with, 80–81; validation related to, 82; verbal aikido practice and, 102–103; words susceptible to, 78–79; worksheet illustrating, 75–77

Hooks metaphor, 72–74

Hooks Worksheet, 75–77

hooky words game, 78–79

I

ideas, holding to lightly, 36–37

importance: assessing away moves relative to, 50–51; determining with clients, 22–23, 33

informed consent, 28, 160

inner experiences: clients claiming to control, 79–80, 81–82; defusing from, 84; exploring futility of controlling, 67–70; five-senses experiences vs., 2; paradoxical effects of controlling, 82–83; sorting five-senses and, 70–72; trap of limiting hooks to, 80–81; verbal aikido and, 97

inner obstacles, 23

inner rule-giver, 123–124

integrative behavioral couples therapy, 251

internal reinforcement, 195

interpersonal behavior: questionnaire for assessing, 163; shaping with verbal aikido for two, 173–176; therapeutic relationship and, 27, 161, 162

intervention success, 244–245

intimate relating: context for learning, 160; definition of, 159–160

JKL

Joy of Parenting, The (Coyne and Murrell), 190

jungle-related metaphor, 188

Kabat-Zinn, Jon, 42

Kazdin, Alan, 190

kindness, 192–193

Koerner, Kelly, 89, 90

language: flexible use of, 37; human social relating and, 158, 159; problems with, 8–9; RFT and, 9–10

learning, present-moment, 15, 27

Learning RFT (Törneke), 9

life coaching, 225–242; examples illustrating, 234–242; getting on track through, 229–231; homework assignments in, 227, 229; hooks considered in, 227–229; introducing the matrix in, 225–227; life purpose and, 225, 226–227, 228, 229; noticing as key to, 242; nurturing environment for, 233; overcoming external barriers through, 231–233; putting people first in, 233–234; sorting process in, 230–231

life stories, 5

Linehan, Marsha, 90

love, 166, 168, 169–170

low-probability behaviors, 194

M

Man in the Hole metaphor, 52–54

Marcus Aurelius, 67

Masks game, 207–208

the matrix, 2–3; ACT integration with, 252–253; awareness, courage, love and, 166–169; behavioral activation and,

248–250; CBT used with, 252; children and, 202–208; clinically relevant behaviors and, 153–154; couples work and, 209–223; definition/description of, 255; deictic framing and, 146; dialectical behavior therapy and, 251–252; functional contextualism and, 35, 153, 243, 253; history of, 3–4; integrative behavioral couples therapy and, 251; introducing to clients, 21–26; life coaching and, 225–242; matrix work without, 153; mindfulness and, 13, 250; motivational interviewing and, 250–251; noticing with, 27; order for presenting, 33; parents and, 184–185; perspective taking using, 182; potential traps using, 30–32; promoting flexible tracking through, 128; psychodynamic approaches and, 252; psychological flexibility and, 151; psychotropic medications and, 246–248; purpose of using, 152; schema therapy and, 250; sharing your own, 152; skills central to using, 19–20; sorting experiences on, 4–5; teenagers and, 198–202; therapeutic relationship and, 27–29, 157–182; value of using, 5–6; verbal aikido and, 20, 87

Matrix Activity Log, 248, 249

Matrix Boxes exercise, 207

Matrix Explorer game, 206

Matrix Life Dashboard, 244–245

Matrix Session Bridging Questionnaire, 176–181

"me noticing" point of view, 24

mechanistic rules, 151

medication assessment, 246–248

mental experiences: five-senses experiences vs., 2; verbal aikido and, 97. See also inner experiences

metaphors: Dancing, 187–188; Hooks, 72–79; jungle-related, 188; Man in the Hole, 52–54; Mother Cat, 114–119; waves, 28, 160

mindfulness, 12–13; definition of, 42; the matrix and, 13, 250; noticing exercise, 42–43

Mindfulness for Two (Wilson), 253

modeling, 204

Mother Cat Exercise, 114–119; benefits of using, 126; broadening the use of, 118–119; dialogue example, 114–117; FAQs related to, 121–122; home practice assignment, 119; potential traps using, 120–121

motivational interviewing, 250–251

Murrell, Amy, 190

N

negative reinforcement, 60

noticing: CRBs, 169; hooks, 79; life coaching and, 242; practicing the skill of, 27, 29–30, 54; settling-in exercise based on, 42–43; toward and away moves, 30, 54; workability, 11–12

Nurture Effect, The (Biglan), 233

nurturing environment, 186, 233

O

observable behavior, 105

observer self, 7, 38

obsessive-compulsive disorder (OCD): away vs. toward moves in, 51–52; sorting exercise for, 72

obstacles, outside vs. inner, 23

Olaz, Fabian, 248

orange belt validation, 91

outside obstacles, 23

Stuck Loop Car exercise, 205

stuck loops: children and, 205; couples and, 212–215; parents and, 186; social, 157–158; uncovering, 49–50

stuck stories, 35–36

SUDs scale, 246–247

suppressing thoughts, 82–83

TUV

task division, 194

teenagers, 198–202; authenticity and validation with, 201–202; keeping it simple with, 198; perspective-taking interview with, 202; presenting home practice to, 201; verbal aikido practiced with, 200–201; visuals used with, 198–200. *See also* children

temporal framing, 61

therapeutic relationship, 27–29, 157–182; awareness, courage, and love in, 166–170; clinically relevant behaviors in, 162–166; five rules of FAP for, 169–170; human social development and, 158–159; interpersonal focus in, 161; learning intimate relating through, 160; Matrix Session Bridging Questionnaire, 176–181; obtaining informed consent for, 28, 160; verbal aikido for two in, 170–176

therapy: agreeing on objectives for, 26–27; bringing under appetitive control, 243–244; considerations about ending, 111, 147; context of choice offered in, 20–21; measuring success of, 244–245

there-then perspective, 139, 140, 141

thoughts: clients claiming to control, 79–80, 81–82; defusing from, 84; paradoxical effects of suppressing, 82–83. *See also* inner experiences

toward moves, 2; appetitive control and, 8; away moves as, 51–52; clinically relevant behaviors as, 164; helping

clients identify, 25–26; home practice of noticing, 30, 54, 137–138; obstacles preventing, 23–24. *See also* away moves

Toyota Kata (Rother), 234

tracking, 57; avoidant, 124; flexible, 109, 125, 128; noticing of hooks and, 85; pliance and, 57–59, 126; promoted by parents, 192; rule following and, 123–124, 125; sorting to promote, 230–231

traps: explaining vs. pointing, 31; Hooks metaphor, 80–81; left-hand side behavior, 55; pathologizing clients, 56; perspective taking, 138–142; self-compassion, 120–121; sorting-related, 31–32; speaking for clients, 54–55; verbal aikido, 104–106

trauma, memories of, 4

Turrell, Sheri, 185

"Under the Hood: Basic Processes Underlying the Matrix" (Schoendorff, Webster, and Polk), 9

unlikely situations, 138

vague situations, 139

validation: couples work and, 223; hooks discussion and, 82; levels of, 90–92; parenting principle of, 190, 196; perspective taking and, 141; teenagers and, 201–202; verbal aikido and, 89–93

valued living, 1

values, 6; conflicts between, 144; relational frame definition of, 61; use and non-use of word, 23; workability related to, 11

verbal aikido, 20, 87–112; ACT and, 110; basics of, 88–95; checklist on, 112; children and, 205; couples work and, 217–220; dialogue examples, 93–94, 98–102; FAQs related to, 106–108; going deeper with, 109–110; home practice of, 104; hooks work using,

102–103; introducing to clients, 95; multiple rounds of, 103–104; potential traps related to, 104–106; practicing the moves of, 98–104; questions for practicing, 96, 97, 106–108; sorting practice, 89; teenagers and, 200–201; therapeutic relationship and, 170–176; validation steps/levels, 89–93; verbal wrestling vs., 93–95; worksheet about, 96–98; "Yes, and" practice, 88–89

verbal aikido for two, 170–176; dialogues illustrating, 171–173, 174–175; shaping interpersonal behavior using, 173–176

Verbal Aikido for Two worksheet, 171

Verbal Aikido Worksheet, 96–98

verbal learning, 12

verbal wrestling, 93–95

visual tools: for children, 203–204; for teenagers, 198–200

W

waves metaphor, 28, 160

Webster, Mark, 4, 146

Wegner, Daniel, 82

"What is important?" question, 5, 22, 33, 157

white belt validation, 91

"Who is important?" question, 5, 22, 33, 157, 159, 198, 225, 256

words: game about hooky, 78–79. *See also* language

workability: of away moves, 41–42, 54; noticing, 11–12; parenting principle of, 190–191; point of view of, 41–42

worksheets: Hooks, 75–77; Matrix Activity Log, 248, 249; Matrix Session Bridging Questionnaire, 176–181; Verbal Aikido, 96–98; Verbal Aikido for Two, 171

XYZ

yellow belt validation, 91

"Yes, and..." stance, 13, 20, 88–89

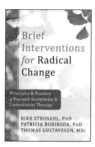
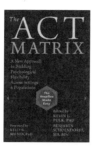
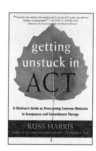
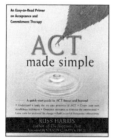
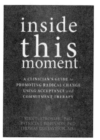
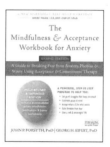

Register your **new harbinger** titles for additional benefits!

When you register your **new harbinger** title—purchased in any format, from any source—you get access to benefits like the following:

- Downloadable accessories like printable worksheets and extra content

- Instructional videos and audio files

- Information about updates, corrections, and new editions

Not every title has accessories, but we're adding new material all the time.

Access free accessories in 3 easy steps:

1. Sign in at NewHarbinger.com (or **register** to create an account).

2. Click on **register a book**. Search for your title and click the **register** button when it appears.

3. Click on the **book cover or title** to go to its details page. Click on **accessories** to view and access files.

That's all there is to it!

If you need help, visit:

NewHarbinger.com/accessories

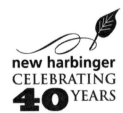

new harbinger
CELEBRATING
40 YEARS